Create the Life You Crave!

HIT THE GROUND RUNNING
PRACTICAL GUIDE
TO ENERGIZE YOUR LIFE

PLUS 12 STORIES OF
TRANSFORMATION & COMMITMENT

LESLIE HAMP

creative catalyst

Author: Leslie Hamp

Book and cover design: Roslyn Nelson

Publisher: Little Big Bay

littlebigbay.com

ISBN 978-0-9834330-1-9

Library of Congress Control Number: 2011925442

The purpose of the book is to educate, inform and enlighten those
persons who wish to explore health and lifestyle options. It is sold
with the understanding that the publisher and author are not
engaged in providing psychological, medical or professional services
through this medium. If such professional advice or service is
required, the services of a competent professional should be sought.

Dedicated to my parents

who shaped my character

molded my spirit

and touched my heart

CREATE THE LIFE YOU CRAVE!

Contents

CREATE THE LIFE YOU CRAVE!

Welcome

Create the Life You Crave!

IN ONLY 90 DAYS
EACH WEEK, you will enjoy an inspirational story,
complete simple action steps,
and read the weekly lesson.
WHAT COULD BE EASIER?

This hit the ground running, practical guide offers you strategies to transform your life – one week at a time. Designed as a 90-day, action-oriented program, each chapter features an inspirational story; simple action steps; and a weekly lesson on one life-altering behavior. With chapters on authenticity, passion, self-care, decluttering and more, you will discover how to assess your current life, identify what's draining your energy and what's feeding your soul, and create a blueprint for change. Frustration and neglect of self will be replaced with momentum, passion and joy.

Read inspiring stories of transformation and commitment by people who have radically shifted priorities, unleashed authenticity, and embraced the practice of extreme self-care.

To begin, buy yourself a beautiful journal because you will be recording the next 90 days of your life. Get ready for some surprises, as you wake up to your unique and wonderful life! Before you begin Week One, take time to answer the Lifestyle Balance Assessment on the next page. Welcome!

BEFORE YOU DO ANYTHING ELSE...
A PERSONAL LIFESTYLE BALANCE ASSESSMENT

Read each statement and score (circle) yourself on a scale of 1-10 (1 = poor, 10 = excellent).

1. I make extreme self care a daily priority.
   1 2 3 4 5 6 7 8 9 10

2. I exercise at least four days per week. 1 2 3 4 5 6 7 8 9 10

3. I take time to declutter my home and office.
   1 2 3 4 5 6 7 8 9 10

4. I write in a journal or keep track of what is important to me.
   1 2 3 4 5 6 7 8 9 10

5. I have many friends with whom I share my hobbies and recreation time. 1 2 3 4 5 6 7 8 9 10

6. I fuel my body with healthy, nutrient-rich foods.
   1 2 3 4 5 6 7 8 9 10

7. I have a family or group of close friends I rely on.
   1 2 3 4 5 6 7 8 9 10

8. I have at least one interest that sparks my energy, creativity and passion. 1 2 3 4 5 6 7 8 9 10

9. I use quiet time to gather my thoughts.
   1 2 3 4 5 6 7 8 9 10

10. I don't get bogged down in unimportant tasks.
    1 2 3 4 5 6 7 8 9 10

11. I am satisfied with the way I balance the commitments in my life. 1 2 3 4 5 6 7 8 9 10

12. I can see the difference between where I am and where I want to be. 1 2 3 4 5 6 7 8 9 10

Total score _____ (You'll be returning to this score at a later date.)

INTRODUCTION: GETTING READY

I just had to let go. Of everything.

"...the year I stepped out of my comfort zone.."

by Leslie Hamp

The year started full of possibility and hope. I had just split from my business partner, patting myself on the back for leaving behind the disappointment and frustration that came with the failed venture. I was back on my own with a handful of consulting clients who were in alignment with my interests and skills. I was leading my all-time favorite 90-day coaching program – *Create the Life Your Crave!* – with 18 amazing women from around the world. And my Pilates and kettlebell classes were flowing with interesting students and positive energy. My life was more than full with creativity, connection and joy.

Then I got a triple whammy of such proportions that it felt like I was standing in front of a fire hose being sprayed full force.

My father was diagnosed with terminal cancer, my mother with terminal Crohn's Disease, and my sister with breast cancer.

In my typically optimistic fashion, I claimed gratitude as my theme for the year, thinking this mantra would keep me grounded during the midst of all the challenges. Little did I know the struggle I was embarking on.

Eight hundred miles is a long way when you have to fly or drive it every few weeks. It was a daylong trek, no matter which way I sliced it. Driving took 12 hours, necessitating an overnight hotel stay. Flying took a full day, what with driving four hours to the airport, another hour to secure parking, two hours for the required security screenings, and the two hour flight.

Despite the long journey to my parents' home, I felt privileged to be able to travel back and forth to help and hold and support and be supported. The simple things... grocery shopping, doctor's appointments, dinner preparation, laundry... all took on new meaning.

Yet the days were draining. I was always distressed to see my mother, now a frail, fragile woman. What had happened to my independent, vibrant Mom? Where was the caring conversation, the laughter, the love?

Top that with the precarious moments spent at the hospital with Dad and the distress we felt over seeing our baby sister lose her hair as she struggled through breast cancer treatment.

It wasn't long before I was overwhelmed and exhausted. The travel, caretaking and emotional stress were taking a toll. Tears were often just below the surface. I dreaded when someone was too nice because it would release the floodgates.

I'd wake in the middle of the night fretting over my work until I learned to listen to my inner voice, which was saying, "Let go, let go. Now is not the time."

When my consulting projects and coaching programs came to an end, it was no surprise that I felt relieved to let these wonderful clients go, relieved to no longer have to worry about being articulate and clever, relieved to give my creative energies a rest.

The only work obligation left was teaching Pilates classes which were near and dear to my heart but difficult to maintain as I didn't know when I'd be home to lead classes or whether I'd have the energy and enthusiasm to inspire others to be fit and healthy.

In the midst of it all, I just had to let go. Of everything.

As I let go to focus on family, I was diligent in taking time for myself. Whether I wanted to or not, I spent 30 minutes each and every day lying flat on a Pilates Reformer machine stretching and strengthening my body, filling my lungs with air, and exhaling all that stress. Such sweet relief.

I focused on daily clutter clearing, purging the mounds of paperwork that accumulated during my absences. I took unused clothing, books and kitchen appliances to the thrift shop. I became ruthless in getting rid of everything that was no longer used or loved, even to the point of putting my home on the market, eager to create space for something new.

And I journaled like no tomorrow – about family, health, gratitude, exhaustion, confusion and overwhelming grief.

It's been a long, tumultuous year, and I am a different person because of it. I'm easier on myself. I've given up the pushing. I've released self-imposed demands that no longer represent me. I am more mindful, taking extra time to look into the eyes of others and listen to their needs and wants. I refuse to get bogged down with endless "to do" lists, new projects and the mountain of life's stuff. I welcome opportunities to be still, to breathe in clean, fresh air, and enjoy the beauty that surrounds me.

This was the year I stepped out of my comfort zone, let go of what was, and mustered up the courage to trust what would be. I allowed the process and feel overwhelming gratitude for the blessings I experienced along the way.

My new mantra? Let go, lighten up, and thrive.

Leslie Hamp: www.lesliehamp.com

GETTING READY

The secret of getting ahead is getting started.
The secret of getting started is breaking your complex
overwhelming tasks into small manageable tasks,
and then starting on the first one.
— *Mark Twain*

90 DAYS: HIT THE GROUND RUNNING WITH 20-20-20

Create the Life You Crave! is simple. Apply the 20-20-20 format and shake things up. The premise is: change one thing, and you'll change everything. Choose days to fit your schedule, and on *each* of those days, apply the 20-20-20 structure, as follows.

20 MINUTES OF MOVEMENT

Move your body, clear your mind! Choose from walking, running, Pilates, strength training or any other form of exercise you *enjoy*. Be sure to add lots of variety.

20 MINUTES OF DECLUTTERING

Clear your clutter, increase your energy! Pick something you can work on for 20 minutes at a time such as organizing your paperwork, deleting unnecessary e-mails, cleaning your kitchen or your closets or your home or office. See how much clutter you can eliminate.

20 MINUTES OF JOURNALING

Write from your heart and keep it private! No editing or worrying about grammar and punctuation. No over thinking. Here are a few prompts to help you get started: *I am feeling... I remember a time when... I'm excited about today because... I want... I need...*

THE NEXT 90 DAYS: HOLDING A MIRROR UP TO YOURSELF

Three tools will become your baseline for the next 90 days.

Self Portrait

Blueprint for Success

Weekly Inventory

WHAT ATTRACTED YOU TO THIS PROGRAM?

_____

_____

_____

_____

SELF PORTRAIT

You have more natural energy when everything is aligned – your environment, health, emotional balance, money and relationships. The Self Portrait worksheet will help you create this alignment.

Answer each question. If true, put a check in the box. Be rigorous – a hard grader. If the statement is sometimes or usually true, please DO NOT check the box until the statement is virtually always true for you.

If the statement does not apply to you, check the box.

If the statement will never be true for you, check the box. You get "credit" for it because it does not apply or will never happen. Feel free to change any statement to fit your situation better.

Add up the number of checked boxes for each section. Transfer those totals to the chart at the end of the Self Portrait worksheet.

Have fun with this! Don't over think your answers or worry about the results. Your responses will help you discover areas that excite you, areas that drain you, and areas that need additional focus.

A. SELF PORTRAIT: HOME AND OFFICE

❏ I can access my personal and/or business papers easily.

❏ I take time to declutter my home and office a little each day.

❏ My appliances and equipment are up to date and working well. (Refrigerator, toaster, snow blower, water heater, toys)

❏ In my closet, I see clean clothes and shoes, stored in an orderly fashion.

❏ There is enough time in each day for all my plans.

❏ My plants and animals are well taken care of with food, water, and love.

❏ I have chosen a home (or apartment) that refects my values back to me.

❏ I don't spend lots of time wishing I lived in another town.

❏ My work and home have plenty of sunny windows and if I live in the north, I have added a "SAD" light to my routine.

❏ My work and home environments feel safe and do not create stress from clutter, lack of privacy, noise, etc.

❏ If something about my home or office is bothering me, I have identified it and have a plan to correct it soon.

❏ My work environment is productive and inspiring.

❏ I consistently reuse and recycle.

❏ I have art and music in my environment.

❏ When I walk into my bedroom at night, it is calm and orderly and the bed is made.

❏ My bed offers good support and my bedroom is dark and not overly warm.

❏ My work space inspires my creativity and productivity.

❏ People often comment on how welcoming my home feels.

❏ Every time I notice clothing or household items that I never use or have outgrown, I put the items in a thrift shop bag and give them to charity.

❑ People are not frustrated with me for being late all the time.

_____ Number of boxes checked (20 max)

B. SELF PORTRAIT: MENTAL & PHYSICAL HEALTH

❑ I try to keep alcohol, sugar, caffeine, white flour and processed foods out of my diet or very limited.

❑ I exercise at least four days per week.

❑ I avoid excessive TV watching and if I have children, I limit their exposure as well.

❑ My cholesterol count and blood pressure are "good" numbers.

❑ I avoid cigarette smoke, and I do not use illegal drugs..

❑ I do not misuse prescribed medications and try for drug free solutions to my problems.

❑ I maintain the health of my eyesight and hearing, with regular medical checkups.

❑ My weight is within my ideal range.

❑ Because I don't procrastinate, I avoid last minute rush and panic and stress with deadlines.

❑ When I wake up in the morning, I usually feel that something good is coming my way.

❑ I don't forget to play, and I take vacations regularly.

❑ I fuel my body with healthy, nutrient-rich foods and clean water.

❑ With trips to the dentist and daily hygiene, I maintain the health of my teeth and gums.

❑ If I find myself having the same negative thinking patterns day after day, I reach out for help in making change.

❑ I have at least one interest that sparks creativity and passion.

❑ I do not allow other people to control my decisions.

❑ I seek out mentors for mental health support.

❑ I use quiet time to gather my thoughts or meditate.

❑ I write in a journal or keep track of what is important to me.

❑ I am satisfied with the way I balance commitments in my life.

_____ Number of boxes checked (20 max)

C. SELF PORTRAIT: FINANCIAL PEACE OF MIND

❑ I have a savings habit that is not a burden to me.

❑ I take care of bill paying and budgeting on a regular basis, instead of letting it become what feels like a huge problem.

❑ My income base is stable and predictable.

❑ I know how much I must have to be financially independent, and I have a plan to get there.

❑ I try not to borrow money but if I have to, my friends and family know that I will repay the debt on schedule.

❑ I try to keep enough money in interest bearing savings to keep my household running for three to six months.

❑ I live on a weekly budget that allows me to save and not suffer.

❑ My tax returns have been filed and all my taxes are paid.

❑ I currently live well, within my means.

❑ The insurance I carry is appropriate and I review my policies every couple of years.

❑ When I plan for the future, it includes a financial plan.

❑ There are no legal issues which will "catch up with me."

❑ I have a will and a living will and I review them every couple of years.

❑ I pay obligations – taxes, child support, and the like – on time.

❑ I invest my money cautiously, without taking risks that are inappropriate for my income or stage in life.

❑ I know how much I am worth.

❑ I am on a career or business track that is or will soon be financially and personally rewarding.

❑ I feel well rewarded financially for the energy I give to my job.

❑ I seek out mentors for financial planning.

❑ My savings will bring me financial independence.

_____ Number of boxes checked (20 max)

D. SELF PORTRAIT: LOVE AND FRIENDSHIP

❑ If I love someone, I tell them.

❑ My family relationships are as stable as I can make them.

❑ I have good relationships with coworkers and clients.

❑ I rarely see someone with whom I do not want to have any contact.

❑ If I find myself drained by a relationship and cannot change it, I am okay with ending it.

❑ I have made amends to people I may have hurt, regardless of who was at fault.

❑ Gossiping does not make me feel good.

❑ My friends like me in spite of what I see as my faults and I feel the same way about them.

❏ I let my friends know how they can make me happy.

❏ I am truthful, but not to the extent that I am blunt and hurtful.

❏ My friends give me as much love as I need.

❏ I do not hold grudges.

❏ My word is good; I understand the word "honor."

❏ When something unsettling happens, I express my discomfort.

❏ I do not have regrets and unresolved feelings about former husbands or wives.

❏ I try hard not to be judgmental.

❏ When a comment has been hurtful, I do not brood over it.

❏ I have someone I can talk to with very personal concerns.

❏ Instead of complaining, I state my needs without whining.

❏ I have friends with whom I enjoy sharing recreational time.

_____ Number of boxes checked (20 max)

SELF PORTRAIT PROGRESS CHART

Record your Self Portrait scores here. Was completing your self portrait an eyeopener? Keep your scores in mind as you develop your Blueprint for Success.

Week #	A	B	C	D
1				

BLUEPRINT FOR SUCCESS

What are the goals you most want to accomplish during this 90-day program? The right goals will inspire you to take action, even if you are shaking in your boots with fear and uncertainty.

FOCUS ON GOALS THAT ARE SMART

Specific, Measurable, Attainable, Realistic, Time-Related

Don't choose goals you've historically chosen but never reached, unless you're in a much better position to reach them now. Leave out anything you think you "should" do. What goals do you want to reach by the end of this program?

Record your goals now and post your *Blueprint for Success* in a prominent place so that you remember your intentions.

BLUEPRINT FOR SUCCESS

HEALTH

MONEY

CAREER

PERSONAL GROWTH

SIGNIFICANT OTHER/ROMANCE

PHYSICAL ENVIRONMENT

FUN & RECREATION

FAMILY & FRIENDS

Congratulations! You've done a lot of work by identifying and clarifying goals. This is an important baseline for the next 90 days.

10 TIPS FOR SUCCESS

As you move forward through the next 90 days, set yourself up for success by embracing the following tips.

1. Commit. Make a firm commitment to achieve your goal. Imagine success, share your dream with others, and develop everyday behavior that becomes the self-fulfilling prophecy to making your dreams and goals a reality.

2. Take one day at a time. Experts agree that it takes about 21 days to change a habit. After just 21 days of the 20-20-20 structure, you'll be well on your way to creating intentional change from the inside out. Start with Day One and take every day as it comes.

3. Think progress, not perfection. Be realistic. There's no point in trying to be perfect. It'll zap your energy, and remove your motivation. Do the best that you can do. If you "fall off the horse" one day, get back on the next. No "beating yourself up" in this program!

4. Create environments for success. Design your environment to shape the thoughts and behaviors you desire, and surround yourself with people who support you along the way. Avoid negative people or those who try to sabotage your efforts.

5. Act like a winner. Successful people distinguish themselves by doing things that are a challenge, things that are beyond their comfort zone. Less successful people take the easy path because they're afraid, impatient, or too set in their ways to try something different. Model yourself after a winner.

6. Affirm yourself. Truly successful people acknowledge and reward little successes along the way. Their attitude is positive and their "self talk" is affirming and empowering. Adopt an affirming mindset.

7. Establish new habits. Changing a habit takes focus, discipline and time. To keep yourself on track, commit to making one change at a time. Think baby steps for the short term, big results for the long run. Think of the 20-20-20 format as a set of new habits you are developing to create the life you crave.

8. Make it fun. If there's no joy in the journey, what's the point? Celebrate your progress and your discoveries. Relax, laugh at yourself, and keep joy as a major component of your lifetime blueprint.

9. Track your progress. Schedule time on your daily calendar to complete the three actions, five days a week, and track your progress. You will gain more momentum by tracking your weekly progress.

10. Don't give up. Realize some days will be easy, some a challenge. Keep going. A habit is formed when any behavior – good or bad – is repeated enough times for it to become automatic. Strive to make the 20-20-20 action steps everyday behavior that creates momentum and feeds your soul.

WEEK ONE: JOURNALING

From fear to freedom

"I had to take back my power."

by Cookie Tuminello

As women many of us struggle with being people pleasers, but for Southern women our worth is measured by it. I think it's a gene we get at birth. Add to that, my full-blooded Italian, Catholic roots and you have a "gotta feel guilty to feel good" double whammy.

Don't get me wrong, I'm very proud of my heritage. I come from a very closely knit, passionate, Italian Catholic family that I dearly love. However, because I was taught to be a nurturer and server from birth, it took me a lot longer (50 years to be exact), to figure out what I wanted and where I was going.

Like many Italian girls, I married early at age 19. Two children and 11 years later, I was divorced, dazed, and feeling like a failure. With a family to support, I got a job and started over. Five years later, I met and married the man of my dreams. After only 14 months of wedded bliss, I unexpectedly became a young widow at 36. Though I was numb with grief, giving up was not an option. Unfortunately, I knew this scenario well. My own mother became a widow at 46.

After several attempts to find my place, I started my own image consulting business. After many years of burying myself in my work and family, I began to question a lot of things in my life.

A friend knew I was struggling and suggested I attend a personal development workshop with her. My life was changed forever. The defining moment for me was when the coach asked me to stop and "check in." I thought he meant the hotel! I had no idea I'd been living my life so cluelessly and unconsciously. I finally got it. And "it" was three powerful revelations.

I had choices.

I had to please myself first before I could please others.

I had to take back my power.

As a result of these amazing revelations, I climbed out of the deep hole I had dug for myself. I became a coach and started my own company at 50. Some of us take a little longer than others to get "it."

After I took that first big step, I thought, "OK, now what?"

The problem with people pleasing is that it's woven into the fabric of your life and into the expectations of others. Once you make the choice to climb out of that deep, dark hole, the universe is going to challenge you every day to see if you're really serious.

Even though I was considered a gutsy Southern lady, people pleasing had diminished me. It had squelched my passion, my power, my purpose, and my dreams. Most importantly, it had taken away my precious freedom.

The time had come for me to reclaim the pieces of myself that I'd given away throughout my life. It was time to take back my power. I started to journal as a way to identify what was holding me back. Every day I would sit in a sacred space and write. It wasn't long before my journaling showed me that:

I was afraid to ask for what I wanted, and

I was afraid to say "NO."

I was afraid to set boundaries.

I was afraid to charge more for my services.

And why was I so afraid?

I journaled some more... about my history, my traditions, and my parents, who had taught me well to be "seen and not heard," "yes ma'am and yes sir." Now I had to risk not being liked.

To illustrate, when I started my coaching business, it was suggested that I use my given name Beverly, because it sounded more professional than Cookie. And of course, believing others knew more than I did, I acquiesced. After about a year, I was having a major identity crisis with the name thing. I had been nicknamed "Cookie" since birth and that's all anyone had ever called me plus I liked it. I decided to risk not being liked. Hence, *Success Source* was born, featuring yours truly, Cookie Tuminello, Success Coach. Ah, I felt whole again. And off I went to claim my place as a successful business woman and help other Southern women do the same.

The good news about climbing out of the people-pleasing hole and up the ladder of success is that the more you apply what you learn, the more you grow and the more confident you become.

I learned that the difference between success and merely surviving was the ability to discover and recognize my own core values (those things I hold most dear), and then integrate them into every aspect of my personal and professional life.

Remember my first two revelations? Well, this brings me to my third revelation: owning the power within.

What a revelation finally waking up and realizing I had all the tools I needed to be successful right inside of me. I just needed to learn how to use them. What a relief! I thought that was a gene I didn't get at birth.

From that moment on, I have dedicated myself to helping other CEOs, executives, managers, teams, and business owners become more confident, more productive, more profitable, delegate more effectively, and create realistic expectations for themselves and their team members. Since then, I've worked with hundreds of private clients, spoken in front of countless groups, and have created my own *Team Up With Cookie Coaching Programs* that every professional needs to know to be successful *now*.

Cookie Tuminello: www.cookietuminello.com

WEEK ONE ACTION

We must never cease from exploration.
And the end of all our exploring will be to arrive
where we began and to know the place for the first time.
– T.S. Eliot

REMEMBER! 5 DAYS THIS WEEK:
20 MINUTES EACH OF MOVEMENT, DECLUTTERING
AND JOURNALING

Take a look at your Blueprint For Success. What one action step would you like to take this week to move forward and why does this step feel important at this time?

_____

_____

_____

If you notice yourself getting in your own way, what will you do?

_____

_____

_____

What are you noticing as a result of taking intentional action?

_____

_____

_____

WEEK ONE KEY TO SUCCESS:
JOURNAL YOUR WAY TO HEALTH, WELLNESS AND CLARITY

The power of the written word is incredible. Whether free writing, making lists or developing full-blown marketing plans, I've seen again and again that writing "it" down will make "it" happen.

Experts say that simply writing down goals and dreams greatly increases the likelihood of actually achieving them. Perhaps it's because your subconscious focuses all of your energy on the goals and dreams written on a piece of paper. Perhaps it's that writing focuses on outcomes and helps you notice opportunities to bring dreams and goals to fruition. Perhaps it's that writing is just a variation on goal setting and has a powerful impact on motivation.

Whatever happens with that stroke of a pen, writing is a powerful way to release stress, acknowledge an intent, focus on an outcome, and clear the path to make your dreams and goals a reality.

A study in the *Journal of the American Medical Association* shows that recording your thoughts about stressful experiences for 20 minutes, three consecutive days per week, can help reduce the symptoms of chronic diseases like asthma and rheumatoid arthritis. The journaling worked when subjects wrote expressive essays, rather than checklists, about their concerns.

In this lesson, you'll learn some journaling techniques that will help you get in touch with your mental, physical and emotional self.

You may have grown up writing in a diary which chronicles your day's events. Journaling goes much deeper than writing in a diary. Journaling is a way to get in touch with your inner thoughts and to release whatever is in your heart. It's about expressing yourself and discovering the magic of the written word – and the magic of your voice and dreams.

THE BENEFITS OF JOURNALING

Increased self-awareness

Increased self-confidence

Lower stress levels

Increased creativity

Increased likelihood to carry dreams and goals to fruition

Writing could be one more tool for achieving self-awareness, growth and success – even for those who hate to write. Whether you are an eager writer or among the reluctant, give this a chance. No one will look at it but you!

KEYS TO JOURNALING

Keep it private. Your journal is a place where you allow all feelings and solutions to surface unrestricted. Keep your writings to yourself, literally.

Get "in the zone." Find a quiet time and space where no one will distract or interrupt you. Close your eyes and breathe – deep inhales and exhales. Leave your work and your worries behind.

Squelch your inner critic. No editing, no worrying about grammar, punctuation, content. No analyzing or overthinking anything. The key is getting your thoughts to your pen and paper.

Keep writing. Write whatever pops into your head. If you think you have nothing to say, write "I have nothing to say. Why am I doing this?" Quickly something new will pop into your head and you'll be writing again.

Use your five senses – sight, taste, touch, sound, and smell – to provide vivid details.

Begin in the moment. Can't start? Describe your immediate surroundings or how you're feeling as a way to jump start your writing.

Be flexible. Keep your journal with you so you can write anywhere. The spontaneity reinforces journaling as an enjoyable activity, rather than a responsibility.

With a little practice and the willingness to face a blank sheet of paper, journaling can become a healthy outlet to get in touch with your inner voice. And if you're feeling stuck or stressed, whether in your professional life or an interpersonal relationship, writing can provide some answers your logical left brain would never allow you to explore.

SIX JOURNALING TECHNIQUES

LIST MAKING

Write 10 things you'd like to accomplish for personal growth and fulfillment. Your list could include anything from exercising four times per week, to learning to paint, to getting a degree.

Pick one item and list three mentors who could help you reach your goal and how they can help. In the case of painting, your list could include someone who could teach you a specific technique, someone who could become a painting partner, someone who could take you to an art supply store.

Trust your intuition, and write for the next five minutes. Read your list, and refine it over the next few months.

Focusing on the outcome, in this case learning to paint, keeps your dreams alive and helps you work toward making those dreams reality. This is a very powerful technique for goal setting both in your personal and professional life.

FREE WRITING

I used to do this with my boys when they were too young to tell me to jump in the lake. Now I use this technique with adults who are curious about proactive journaling techniques. The technique is simple, results powerful. Free writing encourages you to write whatever is in your head.

To get started, write about an item on your list from the first exercise. Pick something that you'd like to accomplish for personal growth and fulfillment and start writing. Trust whatever flows from your mind to your pen. Write vivid descriptions and feelings. If you don't know where to begin, start with that. "I don't know what to write. Why am I doing this? How's this going to help me?" Before you know it, words will begin to flow and you'll discover what really matters to you, deep down.

Write for five minutes.

Reread your words, then write for another five minutes.

Save your musings in your collection of writings. When you look back, you'll be amazed at how many things you wrote about actually came to fruition.

PRESENT TENSE WRITING

Focus on an outcome you'd like to achieve, i.e. being fit and healthy, and write in the present tense, as if it were already a reality. Focusing on the outcome will help you visualize what you want and create the action steps to achieve it.

NONDOMINANT WRITING

Put your pen in your dominant hand and write these words: What do I need? Shift pen to nondominant hand and respond. What's happening here is that you are so focused on writing with your nondominant hand that your mind is not editing what you are writing. You may be surprised at what flows onto the paper.

EARLY MORNING WRITING

The idea here is to write first thing in the morning before your logical brain is awake enough to edit your writing. Before going to sleep, place pen and paper next to your bed. Set your clock 10 to 15 minutes before you would normally get up. When the alarm sounds, grab your pen and paper, sit up in bed and begin writing. You'll likely write: "The light is too bright. Why am I doing this? I want to go back to bed." Resist and write! Early morning writing shows you what's really important. The positive energy you'll experience will carry you through the day – and get you motivated to set and achieve whatever you wrote on that piece of paper.

AFFIRMATION WRITING

Start your day writing a simple statement such as "I will experience incredible success in my job (or life) today" followed by three activities to accomplish that day to take you one step closer to achieving your goal. Perhaps you'll list: master the names of co-workers, develop my own customer service plan, work on team building. Maybe you'll list: buy a new outfit, read about a specific work-related subject, practice meditation. You get the picture. Write affirmative statements to get you to your goal.

Through writing, your subconscious is letting you know what you want or what you need to pay attention to. Make time in your life for this. It is powerful.

ACTION STEP

Pull out your beautiful journal, and practice each of these journaling techniques at least once this week.

WEEK TWO: DECLUTTER

Transforming my life

"I'm confident I can reach all goals."

by Julie Buckles

I felt fat.

I was a writer who wasn't writing.

I felt stuck.

I had made the same New Year's resolutions for the past five years – to lose weight and to write more – and couldn't find a path for achieving those simple goals.

Then I signed on for a three-month *Create the Life You Crave!* workshop with Leslie Hamp. I did not go looking for this workshop. It was a matter of the right e-mail at the right time.

I am not the change-your-life-through-a-workshop kind of gal. I distrust the self-help industry – and quite frankly I like my life a lot.

But I had known Leslie for years, had taken her kettlebells and Pilates courses, and talked with her many times about writing. I trusted her and most importantly I really wanted to move on. I had two young children who had taken over my life but we all seemed ready for me to regain control.

Leslie essentially handed me a tool belt the day we started and continued to fill the tool belt as we went along. Some tools I disregarded and others I took hold of. The one I still pull out often is the decluttering for 20 minutes. I don't use it everyday but I know it's there and that I can start to regain order in just 20 minutes.

More importantly, she listened and didn't just nod her head but kindly did not allow for excuses.

Together we started to build momentum and then one thing after another started to happen.

I lost 17 pounds.

I organized our messy finances – an issue that hadn't even been identified when I started.

I took a part-time position as a reporter.

I taught two workshops.

I built a website.

And then a publisher accepted my manuscript that had been sitting in limbo for years.

I was on a roll and the momentum continues.

I'm taking on more writing jobs, working on the manuscript and maintaining balance with my kids. Leslie never lost sight of the fact that I wanted to be a part-time, stay-at-home mom. She has kids so understands the challenges and joy that come with the territory.

New Year's rolled around this year and the only resolutions I made involved parenting practices. My career and health are in good shape and I'm confident I can reach all goals. I still hear Leslie's voice in my head – and so never allow for the crippling "can'ts" or "it won't work." Because it can and will – one day at a time, and sometime just 20 minutes at a time.

Julie Buckles: www.juliebuckles.com

WEEK TWO ACTION

You can't do anything about the length of your life,
but you can do something about its width and depth.
– Shira Tehrani

REMEMBER! 5 DAYS THIS WEEK:
20 MINUTES EACH OF MOVEMENT, DECLUTTERING AND JOURNALING

Take a look at your Blueprint For Success. What one action step would you like to take this week to move forward and why does this step feel important at this time?

_____

_____

_____

If you notice yourself getting in your own way, what will you do?

_____

_____

_____

What are you noticing as a result of taking intentional action?

_____

_____

_____

WEEK TWO KEY TO SUCCESS: CLEAR YOUR CLUTTER

Clutter. It's everywhere…homes, offices, cars, you name it… and it has the overwhelming effect of robbing us of precious time, energy and happiness. What is clutter?

Anything you no longer use or love

Areas that are untidy or disorganized

Too many things in too small a space

Anything unfinished

Some estimates say Americans lose a full year of their life because of clutter. Is clutter wreaking havoc in your life? Take a quick look around you.

Are you surrounded by more newspapers, magazines, books, mail or e-mail than you know what to do with?

Is it a challenge to find your car keys?

Are your files bursting at the seams?

Are your closets filled with clothing you no longer wear?

Are you often running late because you can't find something you need for the day?

Is it difficult to make decisions or prioritize your business or career goals?

If you answered yes to any of these questions, clutter may be causing untold stress in your life. How you keep your home, closets, drawers, cabinets, office, garage or car is a reflection of who you are on the inside.

CLUTTERED OUTSIDE = CLUTTERED INSIDE

Clearing clutter is one of the most effective personal growth strategies around. Every day I coach clients trying to find ways to increase productivity, balance and enjoyment. As they clarify business, career and personal goals, an interesting phenomenon happens along the way. They clear their clutter – internally and externally.

As they gain more clarity, they eliminate material possessions or relationships that no longer serve them. They create an environment that supports their new business, career and life goals.

Feng Shui experts say that clutter drags your energy down, keeps you held in the past, makes you procrastinate, and creates disharmony. Think about what happens when you put a piece of paper in the pile on your desk, telling yourself you'll deal with it later. As the pile grows, the piece of information gets buried. The next thing you know, you're wasting time looking through the pile for the piece of information. You become frustrated and feel disorganized. The longer you keep clutter, the more it will affect you.

When you get rid of everything that no longer has real meaning for you, you literally feel lighter in body, mind, spirit. You've likely experienced this with spring cleaning or organizing your office.

By eliminating things you no longer love or need, you are creating space for new opportunities, increased productivity and more contentment.

Clearing clutter is not about creating a sterile environment where you eliminate everything. Instead, you'll surround yourself with items that you cherish, items that make you feel good, items that represent the essence of you.

BENEFITS OF DECLUTTERING

Increased energy and better sleep

Clarity and increased creativity

Creation of space for new opportunities

Inner peace and contentment

PLACES TO LOOK FOR CLUTTER

Every room in your house including basement

Drawers, cabinets, bookshelves, refrigerator

Office, desk, filing cabinets and book shelves

Computer and e-mail files

"To do" list that keeps you overwhelmed

Unfinished craft projects

Old photos or anything associated with a bad memory

Unused or broken furniture and exercise equipment

Dirty windows

Car (including trunk of car)

Piles of books, newspapers, magazines, snail mail

Outdated, unused or ill-fitting clothing

All those sample bottles of makeup, shampoo and soaps

ACTION STEP

Identify one area of your life that needs to be decluttered.

Write about how that clutter affects you and why you want to be clutter free.

Create a plan, with timeline, to declutter that area.

Take action! Set a timer for 20 to 30 minutes, and clear the clutter so you can see visible results.

Adopt the following mantra: When in doubt, throw it out!

WEEK THREE: MOVEMENT

How I hate exercise

"These classes are a high point in my week."

by Deb Lewis

I went to my first kettlebells and Pilates classes this morning. The ad for the class promised increased core strength, flexibility and balance. Whoo hoo... Sounds good. Still, I went with some trepidation that I could perform. Could my abused and horribly neglected muscles really be anything but flabby and weak?

I went to my first classes this morning and I dreaded the moment of opening the door... the moment of beginning. How I hate exercise! I never developed a habit of fitness in my youth and my athletic ability can fit into a teaspoon. Would it hurt? Would I embarrass myself? Would my body feel worse? My poor body is unbalanced, weak, and out of shape.

Years of carrying around excess weight and fat have taken their toll on my joints; my ankles, knees, and hips especially. I have felt a slow petrification process subtly taking over me, creating more inertia and inability to keep up with my family. Creeping difficulty bending, pulling myself up easily, balancing, or maintaining stamina. At times, I have been ready to give it up, ready to throw in the towel, to accept my fate as a sedentary person with dingle dangle arms and a jiggle butt. I rebel against the image of trying to be a "body beautiful" person or a "super athlete." Nope, that's not me. I accept myself as I am. Still, I have felt sadder with each passing year about the inevitable loss of my capacity to move, to bend, to pull, or to balance. Becoming fearful of my elderly years and the inevitable falls and dependency facing me if something doesn't change.

So I went to my first kettlebells and Pilates classes. Baby steps... tiny baby steps. I opened the door and there was Leslie Hamp with a big smile of welcome. I picked up the bell, the baby bell, and I rang that bell and I swung that kettlebell through the air and in the ringing of that bell I heard the shattering of the fear and doubt and the rebellious thoughts of inevitable outcomes. And I wrapped the long, blue rubber band around my foot and I lifted that leg and I circled my legs and I breathed in and exhaled loudly, as I rang those bells some more.

I heard the ringing as clear as a carillon. Clanging and dysrythmic at first, smoothing slowly into rhythmic smoother motions, slicing through the layers of doubt, ripping through and drowning out the voice of "I don't know if I can," morphing into "I wonder if I can," sparking into "I hope I can," and then "I think I can."

"Will I see you again?" she asked at the end.

"Yes, six times, at least; the magic number to try something new."

I can!

And I will.

I love the sound of the bells ringing.

More than three months have passed since that first class. Before leaving for holiday break, I turned to Leslie, a huge smile on my face, and said, "These classes are a high point in my week." Now that's transformation!

Deb Lewis: www.bestfriendsmysteries.com

WEEK THREE ACTION

"Plan for the future, because that is where
you are going to spend the rest of your life."
– Mark Twain

REMEMBER! 5 DAYS THIS WEEK:
20 MINUTES EACH OF MOVEMENT, DECLUTTERING
AND JOURNALING

Take a look at your Blueprint For Success. What one action step would you like to take this week to move forward and why does this step feel important at this time?

_____

_____

_____

If you notice yourself getting in your own way, what will you do?

_____

_____

What are you noticing as a result of taking intentional action?

_____

_____

WEEK THREE KEY TO SUCCESS:
MOVE YOUR BODY TO GET HEALTHY AND FIT

Most of us know we look and feel better when we exercise yet many of us still don't make time for it. Trust me; taking the time to move your body will change your life, and it can be simple and satisfying.

The minimum recommendation for aerobic conditioning is 20-30 minutes three times a week. Add another 20-30 minutes three times per week for flexibility and strength training, and you've devoted just 180 minutes or three hours per week. Those three hours will pay dividends again and again. Here are some tips to help you get started.

CARDIOVASCULAR TRAINING

Also called aerobic conditioning, cardiovascular training strengthens your heart, lungs, circulatory system and your mental outlook. Choose from walking, running, biking, cross-country skiing, swimming, elliptical training, kettlebells and dancing. Start slowly, and stay within your targeted heart rate. There are many small heart rate monitors on the market to help you to do just that.

STRENGTH TRAINING

If you want to ensure you can lift a suitcase, carry a grocery bag or perform everyday activities safer and easier, and well into your 60s, 70s and 80s, then strength training is key. Necessary for both men and women and especially for those wanting to shed excess weight, strength training ensures more muscle mass, which increases metabolism, protects the body from injury, and improves daily functioning. Strength training can be done with simple tools like resistance bands and balls, free weights or kettlebells. The key is to work all major muscles groups, as well as supporting muscles, incorporating the concept of repetitions and weight.

FLEXIBILITY

Pilates, yoga and tai chi all result in better flexibility, coordination, balance, and proper alignment. These workouts are popular around the world, so it'll be easy to find classes or one-on-one training. I am totally hooked on Pilates as all exercises utilize deep abdominal muscles and back strength and a minimum number of repetitions to develop core strength and stability. There's not an athlete, sports buff or non-exerciser who can't benefit from developing core strength, which is key to overall fitness and graceful aging.

WANT MORE MOTIVATION?

Here's an article one of my buddies, James Lean, M.D., a psychiatrist in private practice in Washburn, Wisconsin, wrote for me when I was PR/media director of the American Birkebeiner Ski Foundation. It's incredibly motivating, and he's agreed to let me share it with you.

WHEN YOU WANT IT LEAST, YOU NEED IT MOST
– James Lean, M.D.

The next time you feel tired and stressed beyond your limits, try going for a long walk, run or ski. You may find your outing reduces your stress level, improves your mood, and increases your self-esteem.

Though exercise has long been known for being beneficial to one's mental health, it is still an underrated and underutilized "therapy" for those of us who are in pursuit of that elusive quality of "feeling good." If exercise were a new drug it might be touted as a "wonder drug" for our mental health enhancement. It would likely have an expensive advertising campaign behind it and it would be selling very well.

The benefits are great and the side effects are almost entirely positive. The cost is minimal. The numerous benefits to our physical health from modest workouts three or more times weekly have been reported widely and are well accepted throughout the medical community. From lowering blood pressure to lengthening one's life span, regular exercise has been implicated. Perhaps less well known, however, are the mental health benefits that regular exercise can bring about.

We've all heard of runner's high but have you heard of raker's high, shoveler's high, or skier's high? Probably not, but most have felt the exhilarating surge of mood and energy that repetitive motion activities seem to bring.

Intense exercise stimulates the brain to release hormones called endorphins, normally for suppressing sensations of pain and producing a sense of well being. Endorphin production usually begins about 15 to 20 minutes into an exercise session and peaks after about 45 minutes.

Repetitious movements, such as walking, skiing, shoveling and raking also increase levels of serotonin, a brain neurotransmitter. Low levels of serotonin are strongly linked to depression, anxiety and aggressive behavior.

Regular repetitious exercise may act much like an antidepressant drug, enhancing serotonin and bringing about a sense of well being. Like the drug, however, exercise must be taken regularly to maintain its effect.

Other neurotransmitters in the brain – including norepinephrine, another key substance in mood regulation – also are stimulated during exercise. Norepiniphrine is thought to play a direct role in the brain's stress response. Research has shown that exercise increases concentrations of norepinephrine in the locus coeruleus, a brain region that modulates the stress response. Some researchers believe that regular exercise may adjust the responsiveness of the stress reaction system and make it more efficient and better prepared to deal with other life stressors.

"There is now considerable evidence that regular exercise is a viable, cost-effective but underused treatment for mild to moderate depression that compares favorably to individual psychotherapy, group psychotherapy, and cognitive therapy," state Tkachuk and Martin in a June 1999 literature review published in *Professional Psychology: Research and Practice.*

A November 1999 study of 135 college students found that those who exercised frequently were significantly better able to manage high stress. A 1997 study compared 165 women with a battery of psychological tests. Half exercised regularly, half did not. The active women were found to be "psychologically healthier" and "less neurotic."

Exercise is also known to enhance sleep and reduce fatigue. A good workout leaves muscles relaxed and spirit energized. Stress is less likely to bother us. At bedtime we fall asleep more quickly, sleep more soundly and tend to feel better rested in the morning. We likely will feel less fatigued the next day.

Aside from physiological changes regular exercise brings, there are also the more obvious psychological benefits such as providing a sense of mastery over the activity and control in our lives. Self-esteem rises. It also gives us a time-out from the daily grind. Often it just gives us a chance to socialize.

So if you are contemplating entering a ski race or going for a walk, the benefits of a regular workout are more than meets the eye. In fact, your outlook may change considerably once you begin a regular exercise routine.

ACTION STEP

Research and enroll in a class, event or one-on-one training program that will help you get fit and healthy.

WEEK FOUR: SELF CARE

Waking up and living mindfully

"...every thought we think is either health enhancing or disease producing."

by Blake Thomas Brown, D.C.

After many years of practice, every day I wake up in happiness with a smile on my face. Now, it's automatic and just happens.

I grew up in Kansas, and as a Midwesterner, I was doing everything that was expected of me. I had a basketball scholarship to the University of Michigan where I was emulating a medical path modeled by my father and grandfather, both Doctors of Osteopathy.

I quickly discovered this was not where my heart was, so I dropped it all and went into business administration. With my "yearn to learn," I also began exploring Eastern spiritual studies and Tibetan yoga as well as macrobiotic vegetarianism.

It wasn't long before I had an amazing epiphany during a meditation. It was so profound that it completely changed my life as I got in touch with the God in me. I realized that I needed a complete paradigm shift to release my Midwest consciousness, deal with my inner self, suppress my ego, and discover my mission. I needed to find my purpose and start fulfilling that purpose in this lifetime.

I decided it was time to make energetic choices to support where I was, and that meant leaving my business career and company of 10 years as well as the big house, the nice cars, and my marriage. As I made the change, I lost 90% of my friends and family because I was threatening the mores that we had been raised under.

I set out on a path to learn as much as I could to help myself achieve the best chances to be healthy, happy and successful. I moved to California and studied acupuncture, cranial sacral, polarity, reflexology, Bach flowers remedies, homeopathy, Reiki, Aston Patterning, Alexander Technique, Feldenkrais, massage and many other modalities to add to things I was already doing which included meditation, yoga and vegetarianism.

I learned a lot in a short period of time, so much so, I moved from northern California to Santa Barbara to establish my own practice to share what I had learned and what seemed to be working for me and many others. After a few very successful years, my office relocated into a chiropractic clinic and I soon learned there was more to learn. Long story short, I went to chiropractic school at the tender age of 42 and studied numerous non-force techniques that were offered outside of traditional schooling and returned to Santa Barbara to resume a holistic practice with more ammunition.

Over the 36 years I have been practicing holistic health care, I have always recognized the importance of practicing extreme self care. I do so myself and also teach others how to follow the Six Essentials of Life which are how we think, what we eat and drink, how we rest and sleep, breathe, and exercise.

Practicing extreme self care is analogous to extreme skiing. You're at the top of your game. It's challenging. You're out of your comfort zone, and you're committed to honoring your truth. For me, that means personally living and experiencing extreme self care and sharing it with thousands of others.

The biggest challenge is to be in every moment of every moment, which is a bit of what meditation is. I've practiced this concept for

41 years, and it's still a huge challenge to be in the moment and be grateful. Some days are easier than others. For instance, a recent golf game got me totally out of balance within 15 minutes of picking up a club. When I found myself irritated and out of balance, I said, "Halt!" Then I brought myself back to being in the moment and seeing the good and learning the lessons of each moment.

I continually tell others: practice, practice, practice. And that helps me follow the Six Essentials of Life. Here's how I do it.

I wake up every morning thankful for waking up. I think and feel happiness with a smile on my face. Then I spend 20 minutes practicing yoga, doing sit ups, and lifting weights followed by 20 minutes of meditation where I listen to the silence, my breath and verbalizations to self (expressions of gratitude for relationships with Roelanda, my family, friends, master mind group, staff, financial freedom and life style of passionate living that includes spiritual awareness, good food, good wine, sports and travel).

Prior to each meditation, I do what is called the "Power March" where I assume a certain stance and S T R E T C H, holding that stance for 10 seconds on each side while thinking positive thoughts. I repeat this process three times, twice a day minimum. After meditating, I walk at a fast pace for three miles through my neighborhood while I reflect on a daily affirmation.

Affirmations guide my days. On *Good Thoughts Monday* I focus on the positive from morning til night. For *Appreciation Tuesday* I appreciate all that there is and that I have on all levels. On *Good Deeds Wednesday* I focus on small acts of kindness such as buying lunch for someone I don't know, yielding to other drivers or giving up my seat to another. *Thank You Thursday* provides an opportunity to make more eye contact with others as I thank them for their words or actions and give thanks repeatedly throughout the day for everything. *Good Feelings Friday* is a day to express more love and happiness and fill up with good feelings. *Lighten Up Saturday* is a fun-filled, easy and effortless day, and *All Good Sunday* is an opportunity to look at goodness of the past week and week to come. I carry those affirmations through my day, whether at work or play.

I could have retired 15 years ago, but still love to help others unlock their potential, so I continue to work 12 hours per week and teach seminars and do lectures. My office is just minutes from where I live, and I have a fantastic staff supporting me so that I can devote my attention to patients and to teaching others how to do this work.

Each day I make sure my body stays alkaline by eating two to three pieces of fruit, and a green barley product for breakfast. At lunch I juice carrots and enjoy a sprouts-tomato-avocado sandwich on sprouted grain bread, along with my vice – some white and yellow corn chips. Dinner is usually at home and includes vegetables over millet, rice, pasta or a baked potato. All food is organic and most is locally grown and purchased at one of the daily farmer's markets.

While my diet is primarily lacto-ovo vegetarian (raw milk and cheeses, poultry, vegetables and whole grains), I do eat other foods on occasion, especially while traveling in France where I'll always enjoy duck confit and in Holland where I eat paling, smoked eel.

I am heavily into sports still, record all the Kansas basketball games, and watch at a time that is convenient.

I believe every thought we think is either health enhancing or disease producing. As I see it, the health care of the future will treat the whole person, body, mind and spirit and deal at the level of cause and prevention and offer more from a coaching perspective. This is what the work I do now is all about; to make it less necessary for the body to express in sickness, disease and dis-ease.

Waking up and living mindfully is a choice, an ever-processing phenomenon, and an opportunity to be in every moment of every moment and see the good in it, learn the lessons and be forgiving.

Blake Thomas Brown, D.C.

WEEK FOUR ACTION

If a man speaks or acts with a pure thought,
happiness follows him, like a shadow that never leaves him.

– Buddha

REMEMBER! 5 DAYS THIS WEEK:
20 MINUTES EACH OF MOVEMENT, DECLUTTERING
AND JOURNALING

Take a look at your Blueprint For Success. What one action step would you like to take this week to move forward and why does this step feel important at this time?

_____

_____

_____

If you notice yourself getting in your own way, what will you do?

_____

_____

_____

What are you noticing as a result of taking intentional action?

_____

_____

_____

WEEK FOUR KEY TO SUCCESS:
PRACTICE EXTREME SELF CARE

Imagine this scene. It is New Year's Eve and you are alone at the "Center for Rejuvenation and Revitalization." Despite your conviction that you don't have the time or money to waste away in this self-indulgent retreat, you are sinking deeper and deeper into finding relief for that knot between your shoulder blades, the pain in your lower back, your stiff neck... and you are releasing all those self-imposed demands and expectations.

After a day's treatment of gentle walking, stretching, massage and nutritious meals you've only dreamed of in the past, you are calm and mellow. You have an epiphany.

In your quest to leave the details and frenzy of your life behind and launch the new year with a new attitude, you realize it's all up to you and vow to re-create your life with more balance and purpose.

IT'S TIME TO MAKE THIS VISION A REALITY!

Americans get a gold star for being over scheduled, overweight and overwhelmed. You must put self care at the top of your list now. You will be more relaxed, more focused and more available to living your life in the moment and sharing yourself with others – partners, family, friends, coworkers.

BENEFITS OF EXTREME SELF CARE

Your state of well being is more balanced

You become much more attractive and connect more often

Your life becomes less stressful

Opportunities are much more obvious

You are living a life that juices you to the core

TRANSFORM YOUR LIFE WITH A NEW ATTITUDE

Extreme self care results in a healthy attitude. It is about changing how you take care of yourself, how you feel about things, how you respond to life's challenges and opportunities. When your attitudes are healthy, you are more inclined to wonder and question why things happened as they did, how you can do things differently, and how you can learn from the past.

SURROUND YOURSELF WITH BEAUTY

The most mundane activities become luxuries if you turn them into special occasions. Light a candle to transform your dinner table. Drink your tea from a china tea cup or your water from a lovely wineglass. Fill your bathtub with lavender-scented bath bubbles to create a "spa retreat." Pamper yourself with plush bath towels. Fill your office with new life by bringing in a bouquet of roses.

ADD BODY WORK

A massage is a truly wonderful experience, and it may be the only time you give yourself a chance to totally relax and unwind. There are many different types of massage treatments – relaxation, sports, facial and Shiatsu massage, acupuncture, cranio-sacral therapy, and Reiki healing.

Massage or any kind of body treatment performed by a skilled therapist is a superb way to combat the stress of hectic schedules and lifestyles.

Aside from the immediate and obvious benefits of being more relaxed, you'll start noticing other changes in yourself. You may slow your pace, become more mindful, and listen more to your heart's voice. Your muscles may lose their soreness. You just might find yourself with a whole new attitude thanks to the weekly, biweekly or monthly appointment to rejuvenate and revitalize.

ACTION STEP

What does extreme self care mean to you? How can you schedule it into your life on a regular basis?

_____

_____

_____

_____

PUT YOURSELF FIRST

It's common to put others' needs before our own. Now it's time to get selfish – not stingy, but selfish. It is time to honor your highest self. In fact, it is an essential step in attracting success and positive relationships. It takes a selfishness to say "no" when you are asked to help with a project that really doesn't interest you. It takes a selfishness to forego helping someone so that you can get your workout in. It takes a deep self respect to put yourself first and acknowledge that you cannot take care of anyone else until you take care of yourself. If you take care of yourself first, everyone else will be taken care of as well. Trust that. A curious thing happens when you put extreme self care at the top of your list. Others like you more and will be attracted to you. Now is _your_ time for extreme self care.

ACTION STEP

What can you do to be really selfish in a self-honoring way? What changes will you make in your life right now?

_____

_____

_____

_____

_____

WEEK FIVE: NUTRITION

A bracelet kept me focused and fit

"I listened to that inner voice urging me on."

by Kelley Davis

My story began in 2005 after the birth of my second child. Like many mothers, I fell into the everyday routine of taking care of everyone except me. I kept putting on weight, felt depressed, and didn't know what to do.

In 2008, a friend asked if I wanted to enter a local weight loss competition with her. Even though I didn't want to, I knew I needed to do something drastic to shed my excess weight.

It wasn't easy, but I took one baby step at a time and changed my approach to food. I was from a family that promoted a "clean plate" so I had to learn about healthy foods and portion control. I wasn't on a particular program, but every day I journaled what I ate. My mom gave me a booklet that really opened my eyes as it detailed calorie counts and nutritional content. I could see in black and white the good choices and the bad choices I was making, and that totally changed the foods I picked.

In addition to changing what I ate, I added exercise to my life. At first I focused on cardio, walking around our subdivision and up the short hills, huffing and puffing. Then I forced myself to take my workouts to the next level by alternating walking and running. Before I knew it, I could run around the whole subdivision.

I also worked out on the elliptical machine, which was easier because there was no pressure on my knees. I wanted to make sure that I wasn't going to take off just a couple pounds. I wanted to really make my efforts pay off, so I exercised two times per day and did whatever I had to do to get my workouts done, sometimes walking in the dark at 10 p.m.

I figured I had two choices every day – the road where I would eat mindlessly, move little and gain weight or the road where I would exercise and pay attention to what I was eating. The latter makes you feel so much better and is really the only way to achieve long-term success.

When the owner of the gym I went to suggested strength training to increase weight loss and toning, I added that too. I progressed from walking to jogging to elliptical to interval training to stair steppers to weight lifting to kettlebells.

When the scales showed that I had lost more than 39 pounds, I was excited but I still had a long way to go. I wanted to change, to feel alive again, to be a happy person, and be there for my kids and husband. I realized that I could have all the support in the world but I was responsible for making good choices in life.

The truth is, I couldn't look at the mountain of weight I had to lose without becoming overwhelmed. I knew I needed to stay focused and MOTIVATED to continue to lose weight, but how?

I was trudging up a dreaded hill, and my mind was playing tricks on me, saying "Kelley, you'll never get there." The other Kelley was saying, "You can do it, Kelley. Don't give up."

As I struggled up that hill, over and over, with that conversation playing in my head, I had a vision of a bracelet design that would help me stay on track. I tried to find one on the Internet, but there was nothing. I couldn't believe it.

I had my husband create the "Pound Puncher Bracelet" that I had visualized. The bracelet featured numbers on it that represented pounds... 2, 4, 6, 8, and 10. When I lost two pounds, I moved the button over. When I lost four pounds, I moved the button over again and continued that process until I lost 10 pounds.

I knew what those numbers meant. I knew if I wasn't mindful that I wouldn't be able to move that charm over. It was both my encouragement and my reward. With every 10 pounds of weight loss, I'd celebrate the accomplishment and repeat the process until I lost 72 pounds.

The Pound Puncher Bracelet reminded me to make healthy choices when reaching for food. It tracked my weight loss and was my daily reminder to keep going, to *never* give up, and to be proud of the hard work that I had accomplished.

The bracelet is simple and effective, and I wanted to create more so that I could help those struggling on the same path. I knew what the battle was like, and I also knew this bracelet would give others hope and motivation. But I had never created anything like this before and had no business experience.

Still, an inner voice urged me on, and I listened. I was meant to do this and, just like losing weight, took baby steps to reach my goal. I joined up with a company and we redesigned the bracelet. I launched a website, knocked on doors and began selling bracelets online and in a few stores. Doors continue to open with new business opportunities. We now have a patent pending and sell black as well as pink bracelets.

My bracelets are making a difference, and I'm thrilled to know that I was right about my instincts and that I listened to that inner voice urging me on. Every day I hear from others who are experiencing success and making healthy food and exercise choices, thanks to the Pound Puncher Bracelet.

Very few people know my story or how the bracelet helped me conquer the weight loss battle. I wear my bracelet everyday. It reminds me to be PROUD and to stay on the road of health and happiness.

Kelley Davis: www.poundpuncher.com

WEEK FIVE ACTION

As Anne learns: every day is its own new beginning.
Even every hour.

– Anne of Green Gables

REMEMBER! 5 DAYS THIS WEEK:
20 MINUTES EACH OF MOVEMENT, DECLUTTERING
AND JOURNALING

Take a look at your Blueprint For Success. What one action step would you like to take this week to move forward and why does this step feel important at this time?

_____

_____

_____

If you notice yourself getting in your own way, what will you do?

_____

_____

_____

What are you noticing as a result of taking intentional action?

_____

_____

_____

WEEK FIVE KEY TO SUCCESS:
FILL UP ON A HEALTHY, BALANCED DIET

There are so many "diet" books on the market yet Americans are heavier than ever. It's time to get back to the basics. According to the Center for Disease Control and Prevention, there has been a dramatic increase in obesity in the United States from 1985-2009. In 2009, only Colorado and the District of Columbia had a prevalence of obesity less than 20%.

As a FirstLine Therapy Lifestyle Educator, I show others how to reverse years of poor eating habit with the following guidelines. *(NOTE: If you are overweight and have chronic health issues such as high blood pressure, obesity, diabetes, and heart disease, seek medical and nutritional counseling immediately.)*

LOAD UP ON FRUITS AND VEGETABLES (AIM FOR AT LEAST 5 SERVINGS AS A MINIMUM. TARGET 9 SERVINGS DAILY)

Fruits and veggies come in so many shapes, sizes and colors, each nutritious and delicious. The fruits and vegetables that offer the most nutrients are also those of the deepest color, i.e. dark green romaine lettuce vs. pale iceberg.

Delicious, health-promoting vegetables include broccoli, spinach, sweet potato, collards, kale, cabbage, winter squash, carrots, tomatoes, pumpkins and red bell pepper. Delicious, health-promoting fruits include cantaloupe, papaya, watermelon, blueberries, strawberries, boysenberries, kiwi, grapefruit, orange, prunes and dried apricot. Load up!

DRINK UP (AIM FOR SIX-EIGHT GLASSES OF WATER A DAY)

Life and health depend on water. It is needed to carry vital substances to cells, carry waste away from cells, and it's necessary to moisten the lungs and respiratory tract, lubricate the joint surfaces and internal organs and ensure proper digestion. Rather than wait until you are thirsty, keep fresh water nearby as a reminder to take a drink. Add a sprig of mint or a squeeze of lemon or lime for variety.

CHOOSE WHOLE GRAINS AND FLOURS

Whole grains are rich in protein, fiber and essential vitamins and minerals, and they are rapidly converted to usable energy. Refined grains such as white rice or white flour, on the other hand, lose vital substances that nourish us.

Always choose 100% whole grain breads, cereals, flours, pastas and rice that are full of their natural goodness and vitality. Examples include brown rice, whole wheat berries, barley, millet, corn, buckwheat and spelt.

KEEP SUGAR IN CHECK

If you look at food labels, you'll find excessive sugar in just about everything. Instead of relying on white or refined sugars, try using natural sweeteners such as maple syrup, honey, dates or whole cane sugar. They've undergone minimal processing and retain vitamins and minerals needed to metabolize the sugars they contain.

CHECK YOUR OIL

One of the best oils for everyday use is extra-virgin olive oil and the worst is hydrogenated, partially hydrogenated or "trans" fat. The bad fats, which remain solid at room temperature, increase the risk of heart disease while good fats such as olive oil offer a delicious, healthy salad dressing or vegetable drizzle or sauté.

CHOOSE HEALTHIER SOURCES OF PROTEIN

Eating more protein from fish, chicken and vegetable sources like beans and nuts, and eating less red meat and dairy products, is on Dr. Willet's list of healthy eating strategies. He advocates a minimum of 8 grams of protein per 20 pounds of body weight. Chicken, turkey and fish are better options than red meat, and beans, nuts, grains and other sources of protein are even better because they are generally low in saturated fat and high in fiber.

WATCH YOUR PORTION SIZE

Make it a point to add variety, reduce portion size and eat slowly. It takes about 20 minutes for your brain to receive the message that your stomach is satisfied. Chew and enjoy your food, and don't skip meals or snacks. Try serving your meals on a salad size plate to keep portion size in check, and remember that one portion of meat is typically about the size of a deck of cards.

ACTION STEP

Pull out your journal and track your food and water intake for one day. Just eyeball the amounts and record your selections. At the end of the day, review your selections. What did you discover?

WEEK SIX: DO LESS

The voice of cancer

"...I wake up looking forward to every day."

by David Manville

In 2001 I had a personal "911" when I received a diagnosis that rocked my world. Chondrasarcoma, a very rare form of cancer, had set up shop on my vocal chords. I didn't like the invasion one bit as the cancer transformed my bass voice into a squeak. The medical experts told me I'd likely lose my voice permanently.

That's when my wife Terry contacted a physician friend who is an ear, nose and throat specialist. Terry's questions included, "What would you do if this were someone in your family?"

Our friend said that he would see the world expert for this type of cancer and he contacted Dr. Kerry Olson at the Mayo Clinic in Rochester, Minnesota, and told him about my case. A month later we were sitting in Dr. Olson's office talking about my options.

After a detailed medical workup, I received the wonderful news that the medical team would be able to treat the cancer and remove a tracheal tube that I had been living with since my first biopsy surgery, months earlier. Dr. Olson thought he would be able to keep my vocal chords intact. This was good news indeed as my wife and I had no intention of giving up our conversations.

I had heard many dire medical predictions since the initial

diagnosis that turned my world upside down. I had been living with a tracheal tube and was forbidden to swim in our pool but I golfed, kept busy with my two acres of land and garden, and I decided I was going to beat this cancer. I bided my time until my September 13, 2001 surgery date at the Mayo Clinic.

I was scheduled to fly from Detroit to Minneapolis on September 11, 2001. Then the Twin Towers came crashing down, and travel by air came to a halt. But the surgery was meant to happen.

My surgeon had been at a meeting in Denver, Colorado, and, at the last minute, decided to fly back to Minnesota on September 10 rather than on September 11. Terry and I were also scheduled to fly out on September 11, but since no flights were departing, we drove the 628 miles to the Mayo Clinic.

I couldn't believe it. While I was going through a personal medical crisis of massive proportions, our country was experiencing the crisis of 9-11. I remember driving through Chicago; it felt like a ghost town because of the tragic events. Even the historic doors of the Mayo Clinic were temporarily closed – for the first time ever.

My surgery took place on September 13, 2001. My vocal chords were not removed but the cancer was. I was released four days later with a tracheal tube in my throat and the belief that all would be fine. A few weeks later, I flew back to the clinic again, to get the tracheal tube removed. What a sense of freedom that was. At home, minus the trach, the first thing I did was jump into my pool, something I hadn't been able to do in months. It was a gift to feel the water on my skin and throat. I was one happy man.

My incisions healed well and I got a clean bill of health at my twice-yearly checkups at Mayo Clinic. Then Terry and I noticed my voice changing. We knew there was a chance that the cancer could return, as that is common for this form of cancer, but we wanted to be the exception to the 5- to 10-year rule. In 2005, however, the cancer was back.

I was devastated because I thought for sure that I would lose my voice. I wanted to make a recording of myself saying "I do" so that when my only daughter was married, I could answer the question, "Who gives this woman... ?" at her wedding. I don't think I ever told my daughter or my wife that, but if I was going to lose my speech, I wanted those to be my final words.

The good news is that I went back for the same surgery and they were once again able to scrape the cancer off of my vocal chords. The recovery was a lot shorter this time, thanks to some lifestyle changes I had made, including a regimen of vitamin shots from a holistic doctor, herbals in my diet and regular workouts at the gym. I was in shape and determined to beat this cancer.

By trade, I'm a social worker. I'm a teacher. I'm a communicator. And I'm lucky. I still have my voice, and I figure the "big guy" wants it that way for a reason. I still have work to do.

At my last checkup in late 2010, the doctors said things looked good and while I'm not cured, I can live a long time with this form of cancer. It doesn't spread, but it's there and I'm always conscious of it, especially when I eat or drink certain foods. At least once a day, I'm reminded of the cancer when I look in the mirror and see the scars on my throat.

Some people say they're grateful for cancer because it makes them wake up to what's important. I think I knew what was important on many levels, but I did wake up to some big lifestyle changes. I fight the smoking habit on a daily basis. I continue to exercise and bench press 250 pounds at least four or five days a week. I eat organic and natural products, and I take my vitamins and herbs.

Others who know me will tell you I have one of the most positive attitudes of anyone they know. I don't believe in negativity or in dealing with people who drain the life out of you. Really, I don't need the drama, because life is too good.

During the past dozen years I've adopted an entirely new way of looking at life. I know there are things I cannot control, but I can take care of myself by being spiritually, physically and mentally strong. Before I was diagnosed I was only vaguely aware of things such as healthy eating, exercise and spirituality. Now I focus on food and exercise and on my attitude.

I remind myself to keep negative thinking in check and to make the best out of what I have and to enjoy what I can. Terry's take on things is that these medical setbacks have made us stronger.

I beleive that I'm quite healthy now. I'm teaching, advising and working in a career that I love, and I'm digging in my garden, camping, and doing woodwork in my free time. I feel good, and I wake up looking forward to every day.

David Manville

WEEK SIX ACTION

Things which matter most must never be at the mercy of things which matter least.

– Goethe

**REMEMBER! 5 DAYS THIS WEEK:
20 MINUTES EACH OF MOVEMENT, DECLUTTERING
AND JOURNALING**

Take a look at your Blueprint For Success. What one action step would you like to take this week to move forward and why does this step feel important at this time?

_____

_____

_____

If you notice yourself getting in your own way, what will you do?

_____

_____

_____

What are you noticing as a result of taking intentional action?

_____

_____

_____

WEEK SIX KEY TO SUCCESS: DO LESS, ACHIEVE MORE

In today's world, many of us busy ourselves to the point of exhaustion. Many of us give up sleep to do more and more, or can't sleep because of doing too much. Many of us rush here and there trying to do everything, but in the end feel overwhelmed and as if we're actually doing nothing.

Mark Twain said "I can teach anybody how to get what they want out of life. The problem is I can't find anybody who can tell me what they want." The irony of being overly busy is that time seems to go even faster. And even though you are accomplishing a lot, you feel like you are losing ground. You often feel overwhelmed.

10 WAYS TO DEAL WITH FEELING OVERWHELMED

1. **Recognize the challenge.** Feeling overwhelmed is often based upon a belief that there's too much to do and too little time to do it. Where is this feeling coming from? Isolate the cause of your anxiety, take action to resolve it and you'll often discover that you have all the time you need.

2. **Be grateful that you have been presented with the opportunity in front of you.** There is a lesson for you to recognize and an opportunity to determine what's draining you – and whether it's worth all that physical and mental exhaustion.

3. **Accept the fact that you will never, ever be caught up.** It's unlikely you will ever have an empty in-box. There will always be things left to do in all areas of your life. Let it go.

4. **Remember that you can only think about one thing at a time.** When you are overwhelmed, save the multitasking for a different time and just focus on one thing at a time. Clear your clutter.

5. **Be selective in what you take on.** Learn to prioritize based on your core values and how important something is to you. If it's not urgent or important, ditch it. Pursue only what is urgent or important.

6. **Learn to delegate.** You can't do it all. Learn to ask for help and learn to accept it.

7. **Learn to say no.** If you take something on to be a nice person, you may escalate your feeling of overwhelm. Be really clear about what is important to you and live by your own priorities. Always take a day to think about taking on something new, and realize that people understand when you say you're too busy.

8. **Take care of yourself from the inside out.** Eat well, exercise, and practice journaling or stress busting techniques. Then when you have to put in a long day or extra effort, you'll be physically and mentally capable of doing so.

9. **Focus on the task at hand.** Don't worry about everything else that needs to be done. Designate a period of time to work on one task, then another period for the next task. Concentrate on what you are doing rather than what else needs to get done.

10. **Breathe.** Practice deep breathing techniques to relieve stress and release body tension. Take 10 deep breaths to help you stay in the present.

If you're like most of my clients, you were raised to believe that working hard is necessary for success. Yet with so much on your plate, it's difficult to manage and create your life without a frenetic pace. Doing less will actually help you create space to do what you love.

When you are too busy, you simply cannot get what you want out of life because you don't have the time or energy to figure out what it is you want.

If you want to feel like you have more time, simplify. You cannot be everything to everybody. Instead of spreading yourself so thin, spend time to be with yourself. Cut out projects, tasks, responsibilities, shoulds, coulds, wants, goals, habits or routines that are not necessary.

START BY GETTING A HANDLE ON YOUR CURRENT SITUATION. ASK YOURSELF...

Is my life too busy?

Why have I chosen to do so much?

Where am I going with my current lifestyle?

What is it costing me?

Is there a better way?

BENEFITS OF SIMPLIFYING YOUR LIFE

You'll get back in touch with your values and passions, which may not be available when you are too busy.

You'll start to make different choices than those you make on the run.

You'll have a sense of space to grow and come into your own.

You'll begin to practice extreme self care because you see and feel the costs of not doing so.

Do less, achieve more. Be crystal clear, and direct your energy in a specific direction. Know what to take on, what to give up. When you're clear about what you want, you'll naturally eliminate everything that's not related to your goal.

DO LESS AND ACHIEVE MORE WITH INTENTIONAL ACTION

Live by a paper or electronic calendar. It'll help you organize your time and remember those bits and pieces of information you accumulate all day long, i.e. "call Jan." When my sister, mother and I were on the 32nd floor of a hotel in Toronto and the fire alarm went off, my sister said, "Wait. I need to get my Franklin Planner." I laughed and gave her a hard time about it, until I started using one myself. It's like a second brain that helps you prioritize your day into what's really important.

Spend 10 to 15 minutes each morning deciding how you will spend your day. What are your top priorities – a deadline at work, getting your child to an extracurricular activity, getting your workout in for the day, taking a nap? Write it down; make it happen.

Create a personal mission statement. What are your dreams, goals, vision of your future, and definition of success? Use your personal mission statement to define your future. Include professional and personal goals in your mission statement and define action steps to make your dreams a reality. Eliminate everything that doesn't fit with your mission.

Until you take the time to define your mission and what success means to you, it is most likely being defined by others, our culture, the past, wishing or advertising. You'll most likely continue to spin your wheels until you are crystal clear about where you want to go.

When you define your purpose, your mission in life, that purpose provides inner drive and intense fulfillment. It provides certainty in a changing workplace and in our fast changing, uncertain world. Your life's mission is what you can always go back to for reassurance and stability. Take the time to figure out what your mission is. It'll impact every aspect of your life.

And it'll be the basis of simplifying. What is really important to you and your future? How will you do less to achieve more?

ACTION STEP

Permanently cut out three projects, tasks, wants, responsibilities, shoulds, coulds, goals, habits or routines that are not necessary, i.e . things you used to enjoy but have outgrown, volunteer positions that do not directly benefit you, fantasies and unrealistic goals, financial goals that have yet to come true, roles you take too seriously, leadership positions in service organizations.

List three projects you will permanently eliminate:

1. _____

2. _____

3. _____

Now identify your time drains and solutions. For instance, hiring someone to do your filing for four hours, getting your food delivered, using a CPA for taxes, hiring a coach instead of trying to make yourself do something, hiring a housekeeper, seeking help for addictions.

List five tasks that drain you and solutions.

1. _____

2. _____

3. _____

4. _____

5. _____

Now start living in the present! One way to do this is to eliminate your personal "to do" list. Instead of a "to do" list running your life, try some of these options.

Set up a reminder system for birthdays, dinners, social events, and so on.

Delegate. When you think of something that you "have to do," ask yourself if there is another way. Can you delegate?

Be creative. Buy your birthday cards and presents in batches so you are not running to the store at the last minute.

Streamline. Buy groceries in bulk once a month.

Simplify your needs.

List five ways you can accomplish things without being run by a "to do" list.

1. _____

2. _____

3. _____

4. _____

5. _____

WEEK SEVEN: AUTHENTICITY

The red house

"...poems and bears were the center of my life."

by Roslyn Nelson

I call this part of my life "The Red House."

I had moved from a small town to a nearby rural area. The red house was a few years old, on 10 acres of forest at the end of a long driveway. It was modest in size, with a fireplace, a tiny stream and space for a guest. I wanted a break from volunteering, from worrying about small town politics and to create a smaller 'carbon footprint' instead of just talking about it. Here was privacy, black nights with brilliant stars, utter quiet, and views of the forest from every window.

Moving to this house was yet another quest in a life of searching to live life from a deeper place, more true to the values I could articulate and to strengthen those that needed attention.

My first journal entry, in late August, began with: "This will either be a ledger of how to cope with the loss of a cherished idea, or a ledger on how to live with a cherished idea."

On that day, I was struggling to obtain financing. I still owned the house in town that I planned to convert to rental and I owned a small business. My income was not impressive but I had a down payment and a tremendous will to make this real. I had always been able to visualize something and then make it happen. (Beware of what you want...!) The last sentence in that first entry was, "High up in the fluttering leaves of these tall, slender trees is the noise of wind."

As I traveled from bank to bank, searching for loan approval with increasing determination, I also began a softer journey, finding the things inside of me that were resonating with the red house. A photo of myself taken at eight or nine years of age surfaced. In it, I am kneeling next to a fawn who had been sucking on my earlobe. This was a picture of my truest self – being so close to a wild animal, the braids, plaid shirt and jeans, barrettes and look of utter joy. That is the child that the world offered to me and the years took away from me. I knew that I wanted to welcome her home.

The excruciating lending process continued to be a hell, right up to the day before closing. The deal collapsed one day and came back to life the next. I struggled to find financing, congratulated myself for perseverance and never gave up even when I felt the way to be so blocked that it made me physically ill. My own determination surprised me but after the papers were signed, I still felt afraid that someone would come and take it all away. The joy that I thought I would experience after the closing was utterly absent. I couldn't even move in. So, I called my accountant, who I knew did not have fears about money the way I did.

After Lynda reassured me, she told me that perhaps God had a bigger plan for me that I could not see and that she would pray for me. And she did, right then and there, on the phone. She prayed that my fear would go away. She said it was the devil. It was not a word I would have chosen, but I surely knew exactly what she meant. I found her prayer to be so touching and kind, that I thought it may have been the entire reason that I had suffered fear – to feel that love. Since *she* was willing to pray, I thought that I should do the same, but was not sure what to say. So, I gathered, in my hands, the four baggies full of perennial flower seeds I had been collecting, and said aloud, "I don't know where I will plant these seeds." It was my simple-minded attempt to acknowledge that I needed to surrender to the energy on whose waves I love to ride.

So I did move in. I had lots of peace and quiet. I established very close relationships with the deer and bear that visited me. They knew my voice and while respect remained, we lost unnecessary fear of each other. I still follow the lives of a mother bear and her four cubs and think of them as my family. As I write this, they are hibernating, but not together. The cubs, as is normal, separated from their mother and are on their own. The mother is probably nursing a new litter right now and I hope that she remembers to bring them to the red house in the spring, like she did when the first four were tiny.

I started to write more often. I assembled and printed a book of my poetry, then a book of short stories by local authors called "Love Stories of the Bay" and I created more art. I traveled a little, never watched TV, lived through the winters. When people asked, "What's new?" I always had the feeling that something *wonderful* was new but I couldn't remember what it was! I couldn't find words because it was primarily nonverbal; the sense of being here was so nourishing but by the time I might find a way to describe it, conversations had moved on. The play of light, big clouds, poems and bears were the center of my life.

It was surely not all gratitude and musing, however. Many years ago I had a dream where my computer was sitting on a frozen lake and the (authentic) me was swimming beneath the ice. I eventually surfaced through a hole that brought me into summer. Finding that "doorway into summer" is a task I do again and again. Over these few years, I lost many illusions and grieved losses. There were weeks at a time when I felt that I could not go on, when worrying was my core activity and depression was the only feeling I had. The last time this occurred was mid winter. I thought it was about money.

My expectation of selling the house in town had evaporated as the schemes of clever bankers and Wall Street threw the country into recession. The equity in the house in town that I was trying to sell was also evaporating, along with my savings, as I struggled to pay for the house in town and the red house at the same time, all on the income of self employment. All my redundant financial plans which had seemed so safe had become rapidly compromised. I made an escape plan which involved jettisoning both properties and living very modestly. It offered some solace.

I told everyone that I was depressed. I was surprised at how few people took me seriously. During that time, however, I got some very clear messages.

My spiritual advisor reminded me that the love comes back, but not in the ways we expect it to.

A client reminded me that it is important that we don't sleep through life.

A child died that winter and I was still alive.

I read that the author John Kralik heard a voice which said, "Until you learn to be grateful for the things you have, you will not receive the things you want."

I chose the word AWAKE as my guiding word for the new year, and I let my fear go. I wrote a note of thanks to my realtor, not for selling a house and rescuing me from financial peril, but for doing her job so well. I thanked her for who she was. It was a symbolic moment. I was grateful for the things I had.

I'll wager that by the time you are reading this, my house in town will have sold, that I will be publishing a new book of poetry called *Snow on Fire* and that I will be talking, very quietly from the back stoop of the red house, to the new cubs, who will not have much fear either.

Roslyn Nelson: www.glacialdrift.com

WEEK SEVEN ACTION

*Who is more foolish, the child afraid of the dark
or the man afraid of the light?*
– Maurice Freehill

**REMEMBER! 5 DAYS THIS WEEK:
20 MINUTES EACH OF MOVEMENT, DECLUTTERING
AND JOURNALING**

Take a look at your Blueprint For Success. What one action step would you like to take this week to move forward and why does this step feel important at this time?

_____

_____

_____

If you notice yourself getting in your own way, what will you do?

_____

_____

_____

What are you noticing as a result of taking intentional action?

_____

_____

_____

WEEK SEVEN KEY TO SUCCESS:
EMBRACE YOUR AUTHENTIC SELF

If you want to create the life you crave, you must release everything that is not in alignment with your authentic self. You know – those petty or big time annoyances like unpaid bills, debt that makes you lose precious sleep, an overflowing in-box or "to do" list, an overweight or out of shape body, a friend who zaps your energy, a car that breaks down... you get the picture. The list can go on and on. That's why it's time to say, *"Enough is enough!"*

Everything you continue to put up with drains your energy, holds you back from authenticity, makes you irritable, and wears you down in body, mind and spirit. When you say, "Enough is Enough!," you will free your time and energy for things that are in alignment with your authentic self.

OUT-OF-ALIGNMENT PATTERNS

Working too much and/or Not earning enough
Family or relationship stress
Poor self care
Cluttered house, office or computer
No time or energy.

BENEFITS TO EMBRACING YOUR AUTHENTIC SELF

You have more energy to devote to a higher quality of life and activities that excite you. *You stop trying to manage* situations that drain your energy and unnecessarily get in your way. *You grow more quickly* because you are not weighed down with things that are not in alignment with your authentic self.

STEPS TO EMBRACING YOUR AUTHENTIC LIFE

Understand that putting up with things is not useful to you or anyone else and that you are sabotaging your success by tolerating them.

Be willing and committed to living an authentic life.

Stop complaining. Instead, make a strong request of someone (yourself included!) to remove the unacceptable behavior, such as complaining or gossiping.

Allocate money to handle and resolve issues that are draining your energy. For example, set aside the necessary funds to hire a lawn maintenance or housekeeping service.

ACTION STEP

Pull out your journal and create three lists (home, work, self) of 5-10 items that you are tolerating. List anything that is draining your energy and preventing you from creating the life you really want.

POSSIBLE ISSUES IN THE HOME

Geographic location
Size, style, design of house
Walls that need paint
Appliances that need repair
Excessive mortgage or rental payment
Unorganized closets or cabinets
Messy interior or exterior (yard)
Not enough light

POSSIBLE ISSUES IN THE WORKPLACE

Inadequate pay
A difficult or unappreciative boss
Challenging coworkers
Wrong industry/field
Excessive stress
Inadequate training
Unpredictable future
No job satisfaction

POSSIBLE ISSUES RELATING TO SELF

Inadequate self care
Putting everyone before self
Poor communication with loved ones
No spark with significant other
One-way friendships
Poor nutrition
Frumpy hair or clothes
Poor self esteem

BEWARE!

Becoming aware of and articulating items/issues you are tolerating will bring them to the forefront of your mind, and you will naturally start handling, eliminating, growing through and resolving. Sometimes it easier to lump similar items together and eliminate several in one fell swoop. Sometimes working on one item at a time is the easiest way to gain momentum. Sometimes it's easier to buddy up with a friend and motivate each other. Discover what works for you and get on with it! As you eliminate issues that are draining you, jot down specific benefits, results and shifts that happen as you create an authentic life.

WEEK EIGHT: PASSION

Professor writes New York Times bestseller

"My goal is to be able to write for the rest of my life."

by Andrea Cremer

A broken ankle, combined with the simple act of filling in time while convalescing, launched this history professor from Macalester College in St. Paul, Minnesota, to the New York Times bestseller list. Her first book, Nightshade is currently being sold in 22 countries, with editions in 21 different languages. Here's Andrea Cremer's story, in her own words.

I got into writing young adult fiction by virtue of a miraculous accident! After my first year of teaching at Macalester I decided to get back to some of my lifetime loves, which had been sorely neglected while I focused on graduate school. The first on my list was horse-back riding.

The first day out riding my horse spooked when I was leading him from the barn. He jumped and came down on my right foot, crushing it. The break left me on crutches for 12 weeks. With nothing to do but sit, I decided I might as well sit with my laptop and try something I'd always dreamed of: writing a novel.

It was like the universe stepping in and saying 'your life is on the wrong track, you need to write.' Once I started writing I couldn't stop – I'd never loved anything as much as pouring fiction onto a blank page. It made me realize that history and fantasy are two paths that I can bring together on the page.

I was influenced by my studies, specifically the period between 1600 and 1800 when all the persecution of accused witches was going on in Europe. My specialization is in gender, sexuality and violence, so I study witches all the time. I started to think what if the Inquisition and witch trials and burnings that went on all over Europe in the 1500s and 1600s were not just part of human history but were actually overspill from a secret war between witches since the 1400s and is still going on today and only occasionally flares out to affect the society we know.

I knew I needed to find a way to continue writing, so I researched and found an agent. I signed with InkWell Management in New York in March of 2009 and my novel, *Nightshade* sold to Penguin that summer. It deals with the sexual awakening, discovery, and experiences encountered by both women and men in their life journeys. It'll be a trilogy, and I'm writing the other books now.

The feedback to *Nightshade* has been incredible! I'm so grateful to all the people who've read it and taken the time to tell me they love the story and the characters. I receive fan mail (crazy!) every day and I've received letters from readers aged 10 all the way to in their 50s. It's fantastic.

With the conclusion of *Nightshade*, I'm planning to become involved in a new effort involving the "steampunk" genre of science fiction, alternate history and speculative fiction where the universe is one where steam power is still widely used. I see magic and fantasy, mad scientists and alternate history all meeting in an America where the American Revolution did not succeed and a mechanized British

Empire is slowly taking over North America.

In my latest work, which involves knights (offshoots of the Knights Templar) and concerns occult problems in the Europe of the 1400s, I initially thought it was going to be told from the perspective of a young girl who was an initiate into this group of knights, but I realized that there were more characters than just this young girl, whose stories were pivotal and I needed to show what was happening in their lives as well. So I had written about 10,000 words and ended up going back and rewriting the whole thing and knew immediately what I needed to do.

I've come to refer to myself as a "jigsaw puzzle" writer because I don't write chronologically. I write scenes as they jump into my brain and then as more and more scenes develop, I find the ways the plot puts all the pieces together to form the big picture.

I binge write – meaning when an idea takes hold I write for hours neglecting all else in the world. I don't need a particular space or time in which to write. My two requirements are strong coffee and music. I create playlists for all my books that I listen to while writing and while brainstorming plot ideas.

I discovered that it's so important to experiment with different points of view, and that you have to be willing to kill your darlings. That means, cut, cut, cut your writing and be willing to start over. Writing really is rewriting.

I'm having a lot of fun combining history and fantasy. My goal is to be able to write for the rest of my life.

Andrea Cremer: www.andreacremer.com

WEEK EIGHT ACTION

You see things; and you say Why?
But I dream things that never were and I say Why not?
– *George Bernard Shaw*

REMEMBER! 5 DAYS THIS WEEK:
20 MINUTES EACH OF MOVEMENT, DECLUTTERING
AND JOURNALING

Take a look at your Blueprint For Success. What one action step would you like to take this week to move forward and why does this step feel important at this time?

_____

_____

_____

If you notice yourself getting in your own way, what will you do?

_____

_____

_____

What are you noticing as a result of taking intentional action?

_____

_____

_____

WEEK EIGHT KEY TO SUCCESS: DISCOVER YOUR PASSION

When I ask clients to tell me about their passion – what excites them to the core – many are simply unable to respond. Often we just don't take the time to focus on what excites us or what drains us.

This week's lesson will help you get in touch with your passion. We'll start by looking at what motivates you to take action – your personal interests, attitudes and values.

"**What do you want?**" It's an interesting question, and the answer is different for everyone. What you love is determined by your personal interests, attitudes and values which act as hidden motivators – the reason you act the way you do. How you perceive, evaluate and judge events around you are based on your values and interests.

There are six basic values, or passions, that motivate behavior: theoretical, utilitarian, aesthetic, social, individualistic, and traditional. These six values were initially defined in 1931 by Gordon Willard Allport, a Harvard-trained psychologist, and further refined by Bill Bonnstetter, an expert in business education and motivation. By understanding your personal interests, attitudes and values, you will be able to understand what drives you every day.

Theoretical Value – passion for knowledge
Utilitarian Value – passion for utility
Aesthetic Value – passion for beauty and harmony
Social Value – passion for helping others
Individualistic Value – passion for power
Traditional Value – passion for meaning

A PASSION FOR KNOWLEDGE: THE THEORETICAL VALUE

A person with a *Theoretical* drive is concerned with discovering truth – not necessarily spiritual truth – but literal, intellectual truth. Theoretical people tend to work by observation and reason and may be described by others as "intellectual." They have passion for –

Problem solving

Identifying, differentiating, generalizing, systematizing

Intellectual process

Discovery, understanding, ordering

Pursuit of knowledge for the sake of knowing

Tip: When interacting with someone with a passion for knowledge, focus on the rational, analytical and objective nature of issues. A Theoretical person will not respond well to discussing feelings.

A PASSION FOR UTILITY: THE UTILITARIAN VALUE

Utilitarian people are interested in the value of time, resources and money and how they're used. They detest waste, and they want a return on investment. Utilitarian people are motivated by security for themselves and their families. The stereotype of the typical American business person – practical, conservative, status conscious – describes the Utilitarian person. They have passion for –

Practicality in all areas of life

Utilizing resources to accomplish results

Creative application of money and resources

Attaining wealth

Producing goods, materials, services and marketing them for economic gain

Tip: When interacting with someone with a passion for utility, focus on return on investment of time, energy and resources.

A PASSION FOR BEAUTY AND HARMONY: THE AESTHETIC VALUE

An *Aesthetic* person may judge individual experiences from the standpoint of grace, symmetry or fitness, and they enjoy life as a progression of events, with each event to be enjoyed for its own sake. An Aesthetic person is not necessarily an artist but does have a primary interest in the artistic way of life. Such a person likes to be recognized for creativity. Aesthetic people are often good at seeing the big picture and developing creative solutions to problems. They have passion for –

Self realization, self fulfillment and self actualization

Practicality, appreciation and enjoyment of form, harmony and beauty

Enjoyment of all senses

Creative expression: music, writing, film, visual arts, dance

Understanding feelings of self and others

Tip: When interacting with someone with a passion for aesthetics, focus more on subjective things – promoting harmony and personal fulfillment. The Aesthetic person is very much at home with discussing feelings.

A PASSION FOR HELPING OTHERS: THE SOCIAL VALUE

A *Social* person will have an inherent love of people and a desire to see others succeed. Social people tend to place others before themselves and can be kind and sympathetic listeners. The Social person avoids confrontation and can be a selfless leader and team player, and has passion for –

Championing worthy causes

Improving society and eliminating conflict

Seeing and developing the potential in others

Generosity of time, talents and resources

Selflessness

Tip: When interacting with someone with a passion for social values, focus on how their ideas will help others maximize potential. Avoid confrontation.

PASSION FOR POWER: THE INDIVIDUALISTIC VALUE

An *Individualistic* person is motivated by personal power and influencing others. Such people make good leaders, want to be in control of situations, and want responsibility and accountability. Individualistic people will seek to guide their own destinies rather than being directed by others. They have passion for –

Leading others

Achieving

Forming strategic alliances

Planning and carrying out a winning strategy

Tactics and positioning

Tip: When interacting with someone with a passion for power, focus on how a situation can increase their power or advance their position.

A PASSION FOR MEANING: THE TRADITIONAL VALUE

Traditional people are interested in unity and order. They like rules and structure and will usually seek out a code, often a religious system, for living. Traditional people judge others based on their own belief systems. They have passion for –

Finding meaning in life

Pursuit of the divine in life

Converting others to their belief system

Living consistently according to their belief system

Following and dying for a cause

Tip: When interacting with someone with a passion for tradition, focus on an ideal or higher purpose.

ACTION STEP

Identify your top two motivators.

_____

_____

Now that you have an overview of the six core values and know which two are your top motivators, let's look at how you express your passions at work and play. The best way to ensure you are doing what you love is to live by the Passion Pyramid shown here.

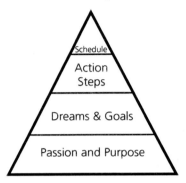

You'll gain momentum and live your passion if you follow four simple steps.

Define your passion and purpose
Define your wildest dreams and goals
Define action steps to accomplish your goals
Schedule time to carry out the action steps

It's not uncommon for people to live their lives from the top of the pyramid down. The result is that they often don't get to their goals and dreams or their passion and purpose.

As you already know, you feel most worthwhile and content when your passion values are being satisfied. The way to gain momentum is to live life starting at the bottom of the pyramid and moving up.

What do you want? You get to choose how you will spend your days. Are you limiting yourself or empowering yourself? What is your passion and purpose? Passion is the ultimate time management tool. When you discover or rediscover your passion, you are on the way to eliminating all the obstacles and fears that have been preventing you from creating a life that excites you to the bones. What are your wildest dreams and goals? Is it time for *you* to live your passion?

When you are passionate, you are incredibly focused, purposeful and determined. Your mind, body and spirit are aligned and moving toward the same goal.

CRITERIA FOR RECOGNIZING YOUR PASSION

You lose track of time when you do it

It makes you want to jump out of bed in the morning

Doing it makes you feel energized and good about yourself

You would do it for free

You love to talk about it to anyone who will listen

You are thrilled to teach others

If you spent all of your time doing this, you would be happy

ACTION STEP

Remember three peak experiences that made you feel totally alive and well – times about which you could say, "That was awesome. I felt totally alive and was thriving in that situation."

Give each experience a title, describe what happened, where you were, whom you were with, and what you were doing. Perhaps it was getting a degree, raising a family, completing an important project, or climbing a mountain. There is no need to spend lots of time contemplating this. Just write down, simply and quickly, the three experiences that popped into your mind. Do it now.

PEAK EXPERIENCE ONE

_____

_____

_____

_____

_____

_____

PEAK EXPERIENCE TWO

_____

_____

_____

_____

_____

_____

_____

PEAK EXPERIENCE THREE

_____

_____

_____

_____

_____

_____

_____

What elements or recurring themes were present in each of your peak experiences? If you listed climbing a mountain, completing a degree, and launching a business, what was the common theme: challenge, learning or risk?

If you listed giving birth, raising a family, being involved in community, was the common thread connecting with others, serving others or being a team player?

ANSWER THESE QUESTIONS NOW

In my peak situations, I felt most alive and engaged when...

_____

_____

_____

_____

_____

_____

_____

In these peak situations, my purpose was...

_____

_____

_____

_____

_____

_____

In these peak situations, I was collaborating with...

_____

_____

_____

_____

_____

_____

In these peak situations, the common theme was...

_____

_____

_____

_____

_____

_____

What if you created a life built around your passions, unique skills, talents and personal interests, attitudes and values? What if you created a life that was clearly the essence of you? What if you created your unique "brand?"

People who create a personal brand appear unique, memorable, soulful. They focus on what they do naturally and others are drawn to them like a magnet.

ACTION STEP

Pull out your beautiful journal, and write about your "ideal" day. Imagine what a day in your life would look like if it were exactly the way you wanted it. Don't just write down what you think is possible – put down the kind of day you'd have if you had complete freedom, unlimited funds and all the skills and support you've ever wished for. Write in the present tense as if it is already happening. Be detailed.

Start with waking up in the morning. Where are you? Do you begin the day with a run on the beach or relaxing over a steaqming cup of coffee? What's your energy level?

Where do you work? (Note: If you are a home manager, mom or dad, describe that.) How many hours a day do you work? Do you have an assistant? Describe which parts of your work are exciting and effortless. Are you managing, analyzing, assisting, coordinating, planning, or executing?

Describe your ideal day in as much detail as possible, how it expresses who you are, how you communicate in one-on-one and group settings, and how you demonstrate flexibility and leadership on the job or at home.

What interactions do you have with people, and who are they? What do you enjoy about them? What are others noticing about you in your IDEAL life? Confidence? Contentment? Playfulness? Inspiration? Leadership?

How do you feel at the end of your work day? Do you have energy to meet friends or your partner for dinner?

How do you take care of your body, mind, and spirit on this ideal day? Describe what your time with family and friends looks like. What support systems do you have in place in this ideal day? A house-cleaning service, a personal chef, an errand-runner? How have you freed up your time to do more of what you LOVE? Remember that you can have anything you want in this ideal day... money is not an issue. Don't hold back. Have fun with this! What do you want your ideal life to LOOK like?

Write your ideal, reread it, and come up with a plan to incorporate the things you wrote about in your current work setting and personal life.

WEEK NINE: STYLE

I remember being scared

"I had the realization: I am a professional artist."

by Gailyn Holmgren

I had a looming deadline. With just three weeks to prepare for my solo art show at the *Art and Invention Gallery* in Nashville, Tennessee, I was beginning to buckle under the pressure of marketing myself. I knew I had quality art and the framed pieces were ready to go, but I couldn't get my head around all the marketing details related to the show. I worried that I would fuss about all of it but have nothing concrete implemented, and that I would look foolish at the reception. I worried that I'd feel regretful that I didn't present my work, and myself, as well as I could have.

Uncertain of the next steps to take, I turned to coaching. I needed a step-by-step action plan that would leave me feeling confident, calm and ready to enjoy my opening, and I knew Leslie could help me wrap my head around everything. She asked me key questions: How did I want my art to be displayed on the walls of the gallery? What did I want to write in my artist statement for each painting? How did I want to present myself and interact with others at the reception? What were my sales goals? In response, Leslie and I developed a step-by-step action plan.

Step 1   Develop gallery contract, including purchaser's reproduction rights.

Step 2   Define categories of art.

Step 3   Develop print materials: an artist statement for each painting and postcards with one of Gailyn's surrealistic images on one side and contact information on the other.

Step 4   Send framed art to gallery owners.

Step 5   Define how to converse with each patron.

Step 6   Visualize the exact outcome desired, from leaving Minneapolis to flying to Nashville to dressing for the reception to conversations with patrons to closing the sale.

Step 7   Celebrate.

When the big day arrived, I was ready. The reception was exactly as I had visualized. I walked into the space and saw my work on every wall. I connected with the gallery owners and patrons and had fun describing my work, discovering what others saw in it, and selling my art for prices that surprised me. For the first time I had the realization that *I am a professional artist* with a gallery representing me. People want to buy my work. That is what all artists want.

Before I knew it, I had closed three sales and boldly set a total of 10 sales as my goal. Within a few short months, my wildest dreams became reality. When I returned to Nashville to pick up my pieces from the art show, 10 pieces had sold, I was invited to send art to two shows next year, and I can count on a solo show next year!

After I got back to my home in Minnesota, two more paintings sold, including one that I had nearly eliminated from final choices for the show. That $1,000 sale showed me that I can earn a profit by expressing myself on canvas. And it sent me back to my easel, ready to make more beautiful art.

Gailyn Holmgren: www.mnartists.org

WEEK NINE ACTION

*There is one thing stronger than all the armies in the world,
and that is an idea whose time has come.*

– Victor Hugo

**REMEMBER! 5 DAYS THIS WEEK:
20 MINUTES EACH OF MOVEMENT, DECLUTTERING
AND JOURNALING**

Take a look at your Blueprint For Success. What one action step would you like to take this week to move forward and why does this step feel important at this time?

_____

_____

_____

If you notice yourself getting in your own way, what will you do?

_____

_____

_____

What are you noticing as a result of taking intentional action?

_____

_____

_____

WEEK NINE KEY TO SUCCESS: COMMUNICATE WITH STYLE

The next exercise will provide insight into what makes you tick so that you can better understand yourself and others. We are looking at four basic styles: dauntless, inspirational, supportive and conscientious. (Note: you may be a combination of two styles, but your goal is to identify your top style.)

You'll also learn how to recognize the styles of family, friends, coworkers and clients and how to transform your interactions by adapting communication to changing environments and people.

Understanding behavior and flexing your own style to better fit with others can create some advantages for you such as helping you avoid or reduce conflict, saving you time working with or through others to get things accomplished, and creating and strengthening important relationships.

ACTION STEP

Review the following styles. Highlight the items that ring true for you. Once you review all the styles, identify which best describes your style – **Dauntless, Inspirational, Supportive or Conscientious.**

DAUNTLESS: THE DECISIVE, DIRECT, TASK-ORIENTED PERSON

Organizing a volunteer charity. Or a corporate takeover. Or a family crisis. Dauntless individuals dive in headfirst as if they alone have the solution. It seems that nothing, including the highest mountain, can deter them. Known as leaders and drivers, Dauntless individuals are challenge oriented and decisive. The key to a good life for them is achieveing, overcoming obstacles, and accomplishing things. Satisfying roles: leading organizations: business, nonprofits, charities and social events.

Are you a high D? You will thrive in a fast-paced, energetic, somewhat chaotic environment. At work or play, you need adventure and challenge. A weekend in a busy city like Chicago, Minneapolis, Manhattan, Seattle, or Hong Kong is just your cup of tea and will inspire you to be even more productive.

GENERAL CHARACTERISTICS

Adventuresome	Competitive	Daring
Decisive	Direct	Innovative
Persistent	Problem solver	Results-oriented
Self starter		

POTENTIAL BLIND SPOT

Impatient	Do not listen well
Quick to anger	Create fear in others
Juggle too much at once	Interrupt
Act or speak before thinking	Takes unecessary risks

INSPIRATIONAL: THE EXPRESSIVE, ENTHUSIASTIC, PEOPLE-ORIENTED PERSON

Social, expressive and full of ideas, Inspirational individuals love a good time and a good audience. They thrive on being where the action is, are fast-paced, energetic and outgoing. The key to a good life for them is building networks of friends who will appreciate their flair for fun and creativity. Good roles: sales, entertainment, public relations, social directors (whether work or play).

Are you a high I? You will thrive in an environment filled with people. Team building, brainstorming, high-energy conventions, or cutting-edge community organizations can send you to amazing new levels of success.

GENERAL CHARACTERISTICS

Charming	Confident	Convincing
Enthusiastic	Inspiring	Optimistic
Persuasive	Popular	Sociable
Trusting	Accurate	Analytical
Conscientious	Courteous	

POTENTIAL BLIND SPOTS

Talk before thinking	Lose track of time
Often late, hurried	Disorganized
Overly optimistic	Abandon position in conflict
Can be superficial	Overly trusting

SUPPORTIVE: THE METHODICAL, RELIABLE AND TEAM-ORIENTED PERSON

Friendly and personable, Supportive individuals are low-key, calm and discreet. These easygoing folks operate at a slow, steady pace and seldom show excessive emotion. The key to a good life for them is being part of an ongoing team (business, social, religious) that proceeds slowly and methodically. Satisfying roles: teaching, ministry, counselors, and customer service.

Are you a high S? You will thrive in a calm and consistent environment. A day walking in the woods or sitting by the water can provide you with the balance and peace you need to get the job done.

GENERAL CHARACTERISTICS

Amiable, friendly	Understanding	Good listener
Patient	Relaxed	Sincere
Team player	Steady, stable	

POTENTIAL BLIND SPOTS

Hold a grudge	Resistant to change
Too indirect when communicating	Too low risk

CONSCIENTIOUS: THE ANALYTICAL, EXACTING, QUALITY-CONSCIOUS PERSON

This person is serious and analytical with long-range goals. These conscientious individuals value efficiency, logic and accuracy. They prefer tasks over people and are cautious, thorough and contemplative. The key to a good life for them is making careful progress.

Satisfying roles: bookkeepers, engineers, computer programmers and architects.

Are you a high C? You will thrive in an environment that is filled with order, facts, structure, and one that focuses on tradition. A day reading a book or gathering new insights at a museum will provide balance and motivation.

GENERAL CHARACTERISTICS

Diplomatic	Fact-finder	High standards
Mature	Patient	Precise

POTENTIAL BLIND SPOTS

Require too much data	Hard on self
Make excessive rules	Too critical of others
Experience analytical paralysis	Cannot take reasonable risks

ACTION STEP

Can you identify your core style? Can you recognize the core style of others? Put yourself on the following list, and identify one person who likely falls into each of the other four behavior styles:

Core D: _____

Core I: _____

Core S: _____

Core C: _____

Pull out your beautiful journal and think about a situation in your life that is causing frustration. Identify and write about the styles of those you are interacting with, their characteristics and potential blind spots. Journal about how you are "flexing" your communication style differently to reduce frustration and increase communication – and how you are turning the interaction into a positive one.

WEEK TEN: STANDARDS

Running across Ethiopia

"...we are connected as brothers and sisters..."

by Hans Voss

During a weekly run, Hans Voss, executive director of the Michigan Land Use Institute *and Chris Treter, owner of* Higher Ground Trading Company *in Traverse City, Michigan, came up with the idea of running 240 miles across Ethiopia to help the town of Afursa Wara, where Treter buys some of the world's most sought-after coffee beans. They formed a new nonprofit,* On the Ground; *teamed up with members of the Ethiopian coffee cooperative,* Oromia; *recruited 10 Americans and six Ethiopian runners for the January 2011 ultra-marathon; and raised more than $100,000 to help build and supply rural schools in Afursa Wara, a region that's considered the poorest of the poor. Here's their story, as told by Hans Voss.*

Today, after 10 days of running, we arrived in Yirgacheffe, our pen-ultimate destination on the Run Across Ethiopia (RAE). There is a real sense of accomplishment shared by the 16 runners (10 Americans and six Ethiopians). We've come a long way together and have overcome some real challenges. It's a momentous point in this rugged journey. After more than a year of visioning, planning, fundraising, training, and then actually nailing the 10 days of running, we are here; we've done it. Yes, there's jubilation and celebration, but for me at least, this is a chance to reflect on what we've experienced and the lessons to be learned.

First, running 240 miles in 10 days, no matter how outrageous it may seem, is totally doable. I am no big time athlete. Most of us on this team are regular folks. We just brought a little extra vision and a commitment to pushing our bodies beyond conventional limits.

For me, this expedition has been especially wonderful because my wife Maureen and my daughters, Aiden and Lucy, joined the RAE team on day six of the run. They've shared the same experiences connecting with the wonderful Ethiopian people, had the same chances to witness the magical African landscape, and they've even logged considerable day-to-day miles running with the team.

This afternoon, after we arrived in Yirgacheffe, my daughters gave me big hugs and sincere congratulations. I told them that this run – in fact this whole effort to raise funds to build schools and support children in Ethiopia – is an example that anything is possible.

What sounded impossible (crazy? unattainable?) is now done. We did it one step at a time, one day at a time, with our eyes on the destination and our focus in the moment. I told my kids that this is just one small example that if you put your mind to something, no matter how daunting, you can do it. I sincerely believe it to be true.

It's a notion that I've tried to incorporate in my life for some time now, but I have to say that this is one of the more powerful testaments to that principle I have ever been a part of.

The biggest lessons though, have come from the Ethiopian people. They are so warm, kind, and genuine. Glowing smiles. Pure joy. So many Ethiopians have cheered us on. There's nothing better than when we run by a small hut in the countryside, those inside notice our presence, and then bolt out with arms waving, eyes wide open, and love in their hearts.

Yesterday, we visited the community where construction has begun on one of the schools the RAE donors have made possible. It was as powerful a human experience as I have ever had: the gratitude of a few thousand people flowing endlessly toward us. Ten runners, a number of crucial role players, and over 700 donors have made a huge impact for thousands of people in this community – and all they wanted to say was thank you.

As I watched their faces, I was struck with how we are much more alike than we are different. Just like us, they work hard, do what they can for their children, and contribute to their community. It does not matter how much we own or how much money we make, what ties us together – what makes us human – is something much more important than that. Frankly, I am not sure exactly what that is, but I know it has something to do with how we reach out to each other with love, no matter how different our cultures may be. That love binds us together. That love is something I believe in.

Voss Equipment is one of the financial sponsors of this run. Voss Equipment is a forklift company that my grandfather, an immigrant from Holland, started in the 1930s, just after the depression. My father dedicated his career to this business and my brother is now the CEO. I raise it because in some respects this business embodies my family story.

It just so happened that I was born into a family that was just one generation removed from Holland. My grandfather and father worked hard to build a business that created real economic opportunity for me. They carved out their piece of the American Dream.

Now, here I am in Ethiopia. Voss Equipment is proudly printed on the back of the official RAE shirts, the same shirts worn by six Ethiopian runners whose family history could not be more different than mine. The same six runners with whom I've struggled with, sweated with, and celebrated with. The same six runners who have shown nothing but kindness and support from day one. It's the same lesson: no matter how far apart we may seem or how different our backgrounds are, we are connected as brothers and sisters on this planet. You just have to see it.

The *Run Across Ethiopia* is an outrageous success. To all the wonderful people who made this happen, I want to say "thank you" and I want you to know that your involvement is making a real difference in the lives of thousands of people.

Hans Voss: www.onthegroundglobal.org

WEEK TEN ACTION

Don't bother just to be better than your contemporaries or predecessors. Try to be better than yourself.

– William Faulkner

REMEMBER! 5 DAYS THIS WEEK:
20 MINUTES EACH OF MOVEMENT, DECLUTTERING AND JOURNALING

Take a look at your Blueprint For Success. What one action step would you like to take this week to move forward and why does this step feel important at this time?

_____

_____

_____

If you notice yourself getting in your own way, what will you do?

_____

_____

_____

What are you noticing as a result of taking intentional action?

_____

_____

_____

WEEK TEN KEY TO SUCCESS: RAISE YOUR STANDARDS

Have you given much thought to how much to expect from yourself and others? These standards are the behaviors and actions which you hold yourself to honoring.

A high personal standard is a choice that will provide you with a higher quality of life. Standards are not affirmations, which are about creating a future that you're trying to grow into. Standards are what is already true. There is very little creation; it's more about articulating what is already true.

Once you set higher standards, you may want family and friends to raise theirs as well. That may happen, it may not. Best to model high personal standards and hope others follow your lead.

When you are intentional about setting and honoring high standards, you may also notice that challenges are easier to overcome.

EXAMPLES OF HIGH PERSONAL STANDARDS:

Being positive in everything you say or do

Being fully responsible for everything (the good, the bad and the ugly) that happens to you or around you

Allowing others to be right

Maintaining a reserve so you're not stretched to the max

BENEFITS OF RAISING PERSONAL STANDARDS

You tolerate less

You are aligned and authentic

"Stuff" you don't want stops coming into your life

TEN STEPS TO RAISING PERSONAL STANDARDS

1. **Make a list of five people you admire**; identify their qualities, natural behaviors and how they handle tough situations. What standards could you raise that would emulate their behavior but still be your very own?

2. **Be mindful that you are constructive** every time you open your mouth, while still saying what you need to say.

3. **Stop gossiping.** Avoid talking about someone who isn't present. Period.

4. **Let go of standards you think you "should" have.** Make a list of the 10 standards you most want and are ready for today.

5. **Understand that standards are a choice**, not a requirement.

6. **Fully respond to everything that happens** in your environment. Assume you had something to do with it. Handle it, and raise your standards so it doesn't happen again.

7. **Create the human bond**, and always put people and relationships ahead of results.

8. **Always put your integrity first**, your needs second, and your wants third.

9. **Always honor the standards of others.**

10. **Always maintain a reserve** of time, money, love and well being.

ACTION STEP
DEFINE ONE STANDARD THAT CAPTURES YOUR
AUTHENTICITY. EXAMPLES:

I am someone who takes extremely good care of myself.

I am someone who has no unresolved issues.

I am someone who lives simply.

I am someone who knows what energizes me and/or drains me.

I am someone who _____

_____

_____

_____

_____

_____

IDENTIFY ONE STANDARD THAT REPRESENTS HOW YOU RELATE TO OTHERS. EXAMPLES:

I am someone who is generous with others.

I am someone who touches every person I come in contact with.

I am someone who is responsible for all that occurs around me.

I am someone who responds fully to the people in my life.

I am someone who _____

_____

_____

IDENTIFY ONE STANDARD THAT REPRESENTS HOW YOU CONDUCT YOURSELF. EXAMPLES:

I am someone who is living my passion and purpose.

I am someone who serves others.

I am someone who lives by values and standards.

I am someone who honors and respects others.

I am someone who _____

_____

_____

WEEK ELEVEN: BOUNDARIES

On a mission

"...I realized I was doing what I was supposed to be doing."

by Kathy Gang, M.D.

There is one thing I know for sure and that is: I am meant do medical mission work. I'm perfectly cut out for it. I travel well, I have an iron stomach, and I can sleep anywhere. After nearly a dozen trips abroad, I can say without hesitation that my work has been good for those I have the privilege to serve as well as good for me.

It all started in 2003 when I decided to go on a service trip to Mexico. I had never traveled with "a mission" or traveled with other adults with whom I was not related. The trip was exciting. We started construction on a small adobe home for a family in Navajoa. The trip was unique in that we spent a lot of time with the people we were serving.

I am a hard worker and enjoyed the labor of building a house, but when people found out I am a family physician, I was invariably asked to listen to someone's lungs or look at a rash. It was exciting to use my old job in a new way.

A year later I traveled to Nepal with a humanitarian organization, Porter's Progress. As we trekked, we spread the word about the important issues facing porters – issues like low pay and lack of health insurance, for example. Again, trekkers and porters alike asked me to give medical advice.

I will never forget holding a mini-clinic in a Buddhist monastery. With permission from the monks, we had set up camp on their lawn. They were so remote that they were rarely able to get to a medical clinic, about a six-hour walk away.

They all had eye and lung issues related to their damp existence behind stonewall. We had a good interpreter to translate as well as to explain important cultural taboos like not touching or stepping over the monks' feet.

Those first two trips – to Navajoa and to Nepal – showed me the importance of medical mission trips, and I was hooked. I wanted more... and the opportunity presented itself in Honduras, where I've traveled for the past eight years.

My winter trips to the mountainous area of Northwest Honduras have been more intentional as I travel with a team to distribute food, clothing and medicine to the people there. Another doctor and I see about 200 people a day in clinics, which are held in schools, farm fields, or under the canopy in the rainforest.

We distribute staples of food, soap, and clothing. We educate about the importance of washing hands, making food with clean water, and having good ventilation to remove smoke from homes.

I came home after the first trip thinking a lot about what just happened. Did our work make a difference? Sure, every trip we find someone, usually a child, who would have died if we hadn't seen him or her and "saved a life," but was that what it was about?

After the fourth trip I realized I was doing what I was supposed to be doing. I was making a difference for the small number of people that I was seeing. I couldn't change the politics or the injustice that poor people in Honduras met each day, but I could try to balance it out with our work. The trip in turn changes my daily life. My experiences help awaken my senses. When I return, I listen better, I see things in more detail and I am thankful for what I have.

Now I can't travel any other way. I've tried. I find myself packing school supplies on regular trips because I know I will find kids who will need them.

I have such a strong sense of who I am now. I get a great sense of well-being and happiness when I am immersed in a culture, using my talents in a way that benefits someone who would ordinarily be forgotten.

Medical mission work is part of me, and my future will include more time balancing work in the States with work abroad. I'm not sure how it will happen, but I know it will.

Kathy Gang, M.D.

WEEK ELEVEN ACTION

*Well, you've got to stand for something
or you'll fall for anything.*

– Country Western song

REMEMBER! 5 DAYS THIS WEEK:
20 MINUTES EACH OF MOVEMENT, DECLUTTERING
AND JOURNALING

Take a look at your Blueprint For Success. What one action step would you like to take this week to move forward and why does this step feel important at this time?

_____

_____

_____

If you notice yourself getting in your own way, what will you do?

_____

_____

_____

What are you noticing as a result of taking intentional action?

_____

_____

_____

WEEK ELEVEN KEY TO SUCCESS: EXTEND YOUR BOUNDARIES

Have you ever thought about your boundaries, those imaginary lines that you draw around yourself? Boundaries help define who you are.

Healthy people set boundaries, which allow plenty of space for them to fulfill needs and bring their best forward. Boundaries allow space to make mistakes and to experiment with new behaviors. Healthy boundaries attract certain people that nourish and celebrate you.

At some point your boundaries become automatic and require no attention on your part. Most people automatically learn, understand and respect your boundaries simply by being around you.

Learning how to set boundaries is key. It takes time, and you'll have to experiment. Be greedy when defining boundaries and adjust to whatever is appropriate to you.

BENEFITS OF EXTENDING YOUR BOUNDARIES

You will attract people who have a similar respect for themselves

You will have more space to grow because no one is crossing your boundaries

Your standards will rise

You will eliminate fear

No one will "walk" all over you

FIVE STEPS TO EXTEND YOUR BOUNDARIES

1. Understand that you need extensive boundaries.

2. Make a list of the 10 new boundaries — things that people may no longer do around you or say to you.

3. Educate others on how to respect your boundaries, and reward and congratulate those who do so.

4. Use this four-step plan of action whenever someone violates

your boundaries: Inform them what they are doing. Request they stop immediately. Demand that they stop. Walk away without any comment.

5. Make a list of 10 ways you are violating others' boundaries and how you will stop violating those boundaries.

BOUNDARIES AROUND YOUR TIME

Time is very important and easily violated. Some areas where this may present a challenge:

You say "yes" when you'd rather say "no."

You are given a new project that causes you stress.

You are appointed head of a committee because no one volunteered – or you volunteered because no one else did.

You are the one everyone turns to for support and advice, even though you're not getting paid for this.

You are the one who gets things done, so everyone gives you their work to do.

BOUNDARIES AROUND YOUR HEART

Most people do not intend to be hurtful in things they say or do, yet sometimes we do get hurt so it is important to decide how you will create boundaries around your heart. The following suggestions may help:

"That is hurtful. Please stop."

"I've been redefining my boundaries, and I want to share with you what is acceptable and what is unacceptable."

"What you just said is inappropriate. Please apologize."

ACTION STEP

Pull out your beautiful journal. Write down three ways you will extend your boundaries.

WEEK TWELVE: CELEBRATION

A flood of insights

*"Can we transform instantaneously?
Yes, when the trigger is dramatic enough."*

by Rex Elleray

In January 2011, the worst floods the region has endured in 37 years displaced thousands of residents in Brisbane, Australia's third largest city. Among those fearing business and personal devastation were Rex and Michaela Elleray. Here is their story, as told by Rex.

A few days into 2011, an area the size of Texas was completely under water in Queensland, Australia. We watched flood peaks of more than 30 feet high and knew this was an economic catastrophe for the country.

Less than a week later, on my wife's birthday, the floods made their way to Brisbane. Near lunchtime, everyone in downtown Brisbane was sent home from his or her office.

With the river at approximately 4.2 metres (13.78 feet) above normal levels, we were expecting it to reach about 5.5 metres (18.04 feet) in the wee hours of the morning and a peak of another metre (3.25 feet) or so at around 4 p.m. on King Tide. We had to move fast to save one of our retail shops, *Michaela's Gifts & Homewares*. We lifted as much stock as possible to as high of shelves as possible and brought a carload of goods home with us.

The next day was grueling. It started at 4:30 in the morning, and we were at the Depot for sandbags two hours later. We loaded the sandbags and tried to take them to the shop but could not get to the site as waters had cut all surrounding access. We returned home to rethink our strategy. The outcome was a return to the flood water's edge later in the day to hitch a lift to our shops in a "tinny," a small aluminum dinghy brought down to the water's edge by a fellow eager to help those in need. Michaela, a friend who works with us, and I boarded the boat for our "tinny" voyage from the water's edge to the shopping centre. I took some really extraordinary photos on my phone.

We reached the shop successfully and moved anything we had not been able to attend to the day before. Computer records and all the electrical trading equipment were removed and the stock all moved up to about 1.2 metres (3.94 feet) above floor level. We had done everything we could reasonably do.

We were on a slight rise completely surrounded by water. We knew if the floods did not exceed the 1974 record that we would escape unscathed and if the flood levels rose further than that, then we had a 50-50 chance of suffering some damage. We were realistic-ally optimistic at this point and hoped that we would be dealing with nuisance value rather than a business wipeout.

When all was said and done, we escaped unscathed by about one metre (39.37 inches). The underground car park flooded but none of the shops flooded. We were back in business three days later amid surrounding chaos.

There's a lot of upside to growing older including the gradual begetting of wisdom when one is standing at the front of the queue. In my case, any gains in cynicism have been more than offset by greater gains in wisdom. Can we transform instantaneously? Yes, when the trigger is dramatic enough.

The personal experience of unsolicited help from complete strangers, the phone calls from customers, from friends, from casual business acquaintances, and from suppliers has literally staggered us. To hear the Lord Mayor ask for volunteers to help clean the mess and find that double the expected number of volunteers turned up; that is inspirational.

The spirit of the people in this city, the courage of the victims and the generosity of the helpers has rolled back the years for me to a time when I viewed the world through rosier glasses than I have of late.

So yes, it is possible to transform ourselves instantaneously, to perhaps see the world with kinder and more tolerant eyes. How about you? Will it take a flood for you? Or could you just make the decision to transform and celebrate life now?

Michaela and I are so grateful. We had an angel on our shoulder.

Rex Elleray: http://www.ellerayconsulting.com

WEEK TWELVE ACTION

Keep knocking, and the joy inside will eventually open
a window and look out to see who's there.
— *Rumi*

REMEMBER! 5 DAYS THIS WEEK:
20 MINUTES EACH OF MOVEMENT, DECLUTTERING
AND JOURNALING

Take a look at your Blueprint For Success. What one action step would you like to take this week to move forward and why does this step feel important at this time?

_____

_____

_____

If you notice yourself getting in your own way, what will you do?

_____

_____

_____

What are you noticing as a result of taking intentional action?

_____

_____

_____

WEEK TWELVE KEY TO SUCCESS: CELEBRATE YOUR LIFE

At this stage of *Create the Life You Crave!* you have created more time, energy and space to live your passion and purpose.

Now it's time to *celebrate* you! Many of us are so busy that we rarely stop to smell the roses. We all have so many things to be grateful for. Think about the small things that make you smile. Is it pushing your toddler on a swing? Is it sharing a laugh with a coworker? Is it going on a hot date with your significant other?

Our lives are full of many small pleasures and special moments. Remember those magic, everyday moments and embrace the joy that surrounds you.

SIMPLE SECRETS TO JOY AND HAPPINESS

1. Your life has purpose, passion and meaning.
2. Your goals are aligned with one another.
3. You accept yourself – unconditionally.
4. You have realistic expectations.
5. You have meaningful relationships.
6. You believe in yourself.
7. You believe in others.
8. You believe in a higher power.
9. You laugh often and at yourself.
10. You keep your family close.
11. You enjoy what you have.
12. You don't confuse "stuff" with success.
13. You keep pen and paper handy.
14. You do what you love.
15. You are positive.
16. You visit your neighbors.

17. You get a good night's sleep.

18. You listen to music.

19. You have a hobby.

20. You feel needed.

21. You don't dwell on conflicts you can't win.

22. You focus on what matters deep to your core.

23. You enjoy the ordinary.

24. You have fun.

25. You read and learn.

26. You know money does not buy happiness.

27. You express your talents at work and at play.

28. You clear your clutter.

29. You say "Enough is enough!"

30. You fuel your body with nutrient-rich food.

31. You add variety to your workouts.

32. You journal your way to health, wellness and clarity.

33. You discover your passion – again and again.

34. You communicate with style.

35. You do less, achieve more.

36. You extend your boundaries.

37. You raise your standards.

38. You practice extreme self care.

39. You celebrate your life.

40. You radiate joy and contentment.

41. You decide the shape and focus of your life.

42. You decide with whom to share your time.

43. You make a difference.

44. You know the best is yet to come.

LISTEN TO THE POETS

"Our deepest fear is not that we are inadequate. Our deepest fear is that we are powerful beyond measure. It is our light, not our darkness that most frightens us. We ask ourselves, Who am I to be brilliant, gorgeous, talented, fabulous? Actually, who are you not to be? You are a child of God. Your playing small does not serve the world. There is nothing enlightened about shrinking so that other people won't feel insecure around you. We are all meant to shine, as children do. We were born to make manifest the glory of God that is within us. It's not just in some of us; it's in everyone. And as we let our own light shine, we unconsciously give other people permission to do the same. As we are liberated from our own fear, our presence automatically liberates others."

– *Marianne Williamson, A Return to Love*

ACTION STEP

Use your new journaling skills and write down some special moments or people for whom you feel grateful.

Had enough writing? Instead, go for a walk and think about some special moments or people for whom you feel grateful.

Capture and celebrate all that is so important and meaningful in your life.

YOUR FINAL ACTION STEP
YOUR PERSONAL LIFESTYLE BALANCE ASSESSMENT

Read each statement and score (circle) yourself on a scale of 1-10 (1 = poor, 10 = excellent). After scoring yourself, compare it with your score on page 3.

1. I make extreme self care a daily priority.
   1 2 3 4 5 6 7 8 9 10

2. I exercise at least four days per week. 1 2 3 4 5 6 7 8 9 10

3. I take time to declutter my home and office.
   1 2 3 4 5 6 7 8 9 10

4. I write in a journal or keep track of what is important to me.
   1 2 3 4 5 6 7 8 9 10

5. I have many friends with whom I share my hobbies and recreation time. 1 2 3 4 5 6 7 8 9 10

6. I fuel my body with healthy, nutrient-rich foods.
   1 2 3 4 5 6 7 8 9 10

7. I have a family or group of close friends I rely on.
   1 2 3 4 5 6 7 8 9 10

8. I have at least one interest that sparks my energy, creativity and passion. 1 2 3 4 5 6 7 8 9 10

9. I use quiet time to gather my thoughts.
   1 2 3 4 5 6 7 8 9 10

10. I don't get bogged down in unimportant tasks.
    1 2 3 4 5 6 7 8 9 10

11. I am satisfied with the way I balance the commitments in my life. 1 2 3 4 5 6 7 8 9 10

12. I can see the difference between where I am and where I want to be. 1 2 3 4 5 6 7 8 9 10

What's your total score now? _____

NOW! COMPLETE THE SELF PORTRAIT (AGAIN) BEGINNING ON PAGE 10 AND COMPARE YOUR FIRST SCORE WITH WEEK TWELVE

Are you surprised at how different the questions feel to you now and how much change was reflected in your answers? This is an exercise that you can repeat in the future and use as a yardstick for your growth.

Week #	A	B	C	D
1				
12				

CONGRATULATIONS! YOU DID IT

You completed the program. Continue using these simple tools to *create the life you crave.*

Celebrate your brilliance, your talents, your passion – no more holding back. Your goal was to transform your life. You are well on your way. My hope for you is that you continue on this journey and find more love, joy and success than you ever dreamed possible.

Embrace the journey.

Leslie

Leslie Hamp, Creative Catalyst
www.lesliehamp.com

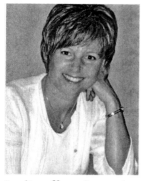 Leslie Hamp, author of *Create the Life You Crave*, lives on the shores of Lake Superior where she enjoys hiking, biking, skiing and kayaking. She teaches Pilates, kettle-bells and journaling workshops and helps entrepreneurs and creative souls establish healthy, balanced lives filled with prosperity.

Leslie offers dynamic programs, workshops, classes, and retreats guaranteed to help others unleash momentum and success. Her book is available on Amazon.com and at bookstores.

Contact her at www.lesliehamp.com

1. physical   6
2. emotional   3
3. environmental   5
4. mental   4
5. spiritual   5
6. recreation/fun   6
7. relationships   6 — kids
8. work/money   6

go for walks

my wish...

my kids would make better choices so I could not worry so much.

(NOT STRESSED)

1= NO SUPPORT   10 Great

my family my job

CPSIA information can be obtained
at www.ICGtesting.com
Printed in the USA
FFOW05n1613130315